Praise for *Longing for Motherhood*

I have known Chelsea for most of her life. I am thrilled that she has chosen to share her story with a view to helping others who walk the road of childlessness. This is not a book of platitudes, but a realistic picture of the pain, anguish, and deep sorrow of being unable to bear a child. The darkness of the valley is real. Having walked the valley, Chelsea points to the hope that is found in the understanding arms of Jesus. I highly recommend this book not only for women who walk this road, but for pastors and other church leaders who want to have a positive ministry to this part of God's family.

GARY D. CHAPMAN
Author of *The 5 Love Languages*

Children are a gift of the Lord, and a good gift indeed. But God does not give every gift to all people. In offering practical and biblical ways for churches and individuals to support, comfort, and even celebrate the childless among us, *Longing for Motherhood* is also a gift. This book reminds us that the childless are part of God's family, too.

KAREN SWALLOW PRIOR
Author of *Booked: Literature in the Soul of Me* and *Fierce Convictions—The Extraordinary Life of Hannah More: Poet, Reformer, Abolitionist*

Longing for Motherhood is a remarkably honest book filled with hope. Through her personal story, Chelsea articulates the pain so many childless women experience and she offers practical ways both individuals and the church can help.

SEAN MCDOWELL
Biola University professor, speaker, author

I'm so grateful that Chelsea has shared her story with candor, clarity, and care for her reader. This book is a balm for those experiencing the loss of a dream and needing reminders of God's great, personal care. Whether or not childlessness is your particular story, may you find reminders of the goodness of God throughout these pages.

KATELYN BEATY
Editor at large for *Christianity*
Author of *A Woman's Place*

The spirit of Hannah is strong in ⸻ ⸻ical—and deeply personal—exploration of ⸻ contribution to the church. Too often, godly women suffer in silence as they deal with this issue. Sobolik's testimony as a young woman will encourage her readers; her relentless focus on God, and the goodness of all that God does, will put steel in the spine. This is a richly moving, brave, and very edifying work, all of it grounded in a beautiful vision of biblical womanhood.

OWEN STRACHAN
Author, *Risky Gospel* and *The Grand Design: Male and Female He Made Them*
Theology professor, Midwestern Baptist Theological Seminary

God will use this book to bring healing and hope to many. Its honesty is very refreshing. In the midst of her own sorrow, pain, and lots of questions—many still unanswered—Chelsea points us again and again to the God who heals our souls, shows Himself mighty and worthy of our trust, no matter what we may face in this life. I am so grateful she has shared her story with us. Of one thing I am certain: I will share this book again and again.

DANIEL L. AKIN
President, Southeastern Baptist Theological Seminary

This is an unflinching, yet moving exploration of the grief and hope that lie at the heart of childlessness. Chelsea Patterson Sobolik helps us look through grief and frustration to see the possibility of a life of true gladness. There is nothing easy about *Longing for Motherhood*—but there is much that is good. Anyone facing infertility or who knows someone facing infertility will find sound guidance here. Pick up and read.

MATTHEW LEE ANDERSON
Writer and Founder of Mere Orthodoxy

I praise God for the gift of faith He's given Chelsea as she's walked the hard road of childlessness. Her resolve to follow hard after Christ in this trial fills the pages of this beautiful book. I know *Longing for Motherhood* will bless many women who are walking the same hard road, helping them grieve well and cling to hope in Jesus, the One who perfectly fulfills all our longings by giving us Himself.

KRISTEN WETHERELL
Coauthor of *Hope When It Hurts: Biblical Reflections to Help You Grasp God's Purpose in Your Suffering*

"I begged Him to remove my weakness, but He used it to draw me closer to Himself." With this honest confession, Chelsea Patterson Sobolik captures both the raw sorrow and Christ-infused hope of *Longing for Motherhood*. Detailing her own journey of childlessness, Sobolik manages to walk the line between grief and hope, confusion and trust, suffering and grace. Her message will undoubtedly be a balm to many an aching heart, as well as a word of wisdom to the communities that surround them, which is why I plan on recommending this book to both.

SHARON HODDE MILLER
Author of *Free of Me: Why Life Is Better When It's Not about You*

Longing for Motherhood is nothing short of a service to the souls of women like me who are childless in the traditional sense of the term. For Christian women who are barren, married late in life, or never marry at all, Chelsea Patterson Sobolik bravely plumbs the depths many of us reserve for aching hours of secret grief. If you've ever wondered how your life can be a fertile, fruitful vessel of expectant joy even as the longing for motherhood goes unfulfilled, this book is a gift for your soul.

CARMEN LABERGE
Author of *Speak the Truth*
Host of *Connecting Faith* radio show

In *Longing for Motherhood* Chelsea offers profoundly personal reflections on the struggles and sorrows of childlessness. This book is not only unique because of the subject it addresses, but more importantly, because of the Savior she calls the readers to cling to. Jesus Christ is the only lasting hope for the hurting.

MATTHEW Z. CAPPS
Senior Pastor, Fairview Baptist Church, Apex, NC

Few understand the crushing weight of childlessness and its lingering pain and sorrow. Fewer still have the courage to share about their struggles in such a poignant and beautiful way as Chelsea does. Her journey as an adopted Romanian child walking through the difficult reality of her own infertility is one of strength and grace. You should read this book, not only so you can see in Chelsea an example of faith in Christ, but so you can help bear the burdens of those who struggle with infertility. This is a resource you will want to linger over and then give liberally to others.

DANIEL DARLING
Vice President of Communications for ERLC
Author of *No Matter How Small*

Longing for Motherhood is a faithful, beautiful, and emotionally moving book. In it, Chelsea Patterson Sobolik draws upon God's character and promises to give hope to women struggling with the trial of childlessness. Highly recommended not only for women, but for husbands, parents, pastors, counselors, and friends.

BRUCE RILEY ASHFORD
Provost and Professor of Theology & Culture, Southeastern Baptist Theological Seminary

This priceless testimony of Chelsea Patterson Sobolik was wrung from an anguished heart, bathed in the grace of Christ, and illuminated by the leadership of the Holy Spirit. Thousands face this or a similar dilemma. May the truths Chelsea discovered be yours also as you read these pages and see that the God of all the earth has a marvelous purpose for all.

PAIGE PATTERSON
President, Southwestern Baptist Theological Seminary

Chelsea Patterson Sobolik pens an intensely personal and biblically grounded account of childlessness. Her extraordinary story is riveting but at every turn she uses her experience to direct the reader to consider the mercy and purposes of God. In a time of such confusion about human sexuality, the nature of the family, and the roles of men and women, this timely and brisk read will leave any reader— whether grieving or joyful, lonely or comforted by family—with a place to start and a vision of God's redemption in the midst of sorrow and suffering.

ANNE KENNEDY
Author and blogger

In *Longing for Motherhood*, Chelsea Patterson Sobolik displays remarkable empathy and grace as she reflects on the difficult topic of childlessness. Through her personal journey, she encourages each of us to refuse the instinct to stifle lament, but rather, to trust God in the midst of it.

SCOTT JAMES
Pediatric physician and author of *The Littlest Watchman*, *The Expected One*, and *Mission Accomplished*

Chelsea Patterson writes with clear eyes and an open heart. As one who has lived through the pain of childlessness, she communicates the heartbreak and turmoil with authenticity. Ultimately, her ruminations on God's role in the lives of the childless and practical thoughts on how to both cope and thrive give her book a hopeful verve that will inspire the reader toward something more than empathy or commiseration. *Longing for Motherhood* inspires a hopeful sense of purpose.

RICHARD CLARK
Host of "The Calling" and Director of Editorial Development for *Christianity Today Pastors*

Chelsea's honest words about her journey with childlessness touched the depths of my soul. Through these pages, she shares personal stories, honest emotions, and meaningful encouragement, all grounded in Scripture. I recommend this book to anyone who has been touched by childlessness, or knows anyone who has!

LAUREN GREEN MCAFEE
Corporate Ambassador for Hobby Lobby and author of *Only One Life*

LONGING
FOR MOTHERHOOD

Holding On to Hope
in the Midst of Childlessness

Chelsea Patterson Sobolik

MOODY PUBLISHERS
CHICAGO

Edited by Amanda Cleary Eastep
Interior Design: Ragont Design
Author photo: robertmatthewsphoto.com
Cover Design: Connie Gabbert Design and Illustration
Cover photo of wild rose copyright © 2017 by Marta Leo / Shutterstock (489204847). All rights reserved.

ISBN: 978-0-8024-1612-4

We hope you enjoy this book from Moody Publishers. Our goal is to provide high-quality, thought-provoking books and products that connect truth to your real needs and challenges. For more information on other books and products written and produced from a biblical perspective, go to www.moodypublishers.com or write to:

Moody Publishers
820 N. LaSalle Boulevard
Chicago, IL 60610

1 3 5 7 9 10 8 6 4 2

Printed in the United States of America

For Michael, my husband.
Thank you for being my David—a man after
God's own heart. I adore you.

For my parents, Bobby and Christie Patterson.
You have given me more than words could
possibly convey, and I am eternally grateful.

CONTENTS

Foreword   11

Introduction   17

1. THE SILENT STRUGGLE
   Why Childlessness Can Feel Lonely   23

2. SEASONS OF SORROW
   What Do You Do in the Midst of Sorrow?   49

3. TRUSTING GOD'S NO
   God's Care in the Midst of Suffering   71

4. GRIEVING YOUR UNFULFILLED DESIRE
   Childless Women Who Found Hope   95

5. WE HAVE THIS HOPE!
   What Does Real Hope Look Like?   115

6. WAYS TO LIVE OUT THE LONGING
   How You Can Still Be a Mother   135

7. DON'T WASTE YOUR CHILDLESSNESS
   Use Your Suffering to Serve Others   155

8. HOW OUR COMMUNITIES CAN LOVE US WELL
   Equipping the Church to Care for the Childless   169

A Final Note   187

Prayers of Longing and Hope   189

30 Scriptures to Sustain You in the Midst of Childlessness   195

Notes   203

Recommended Resources   209

Acknowledgments   211

FOREWORD

*B*efore facing the possibility of never having children, I had all the answers on God's sovereignty and human suffering. I remember, as a very young man, brashly dismissing the atheist objection to the "problem of evil" by saying, "There is no problem of evil. God is God, and He can do with His creation as He wills." My doctrine of God's lordship over all things was correct, taught in, among other places, the apostle Paul's letter to the church at Rome. I was right that many times humanity attempts to put God on trial—"in the dock," in the words of C. S. Lewis—rather than bowing in worship before Him.

What I missed, though, was the way the same apostolic word spoke of the "groaning"—sometimes with utterances "too deep for words"—that comes as we walk through a fallen world, a world that is not the way it is supposed to be (Rom. 8:18–26). I failed to see the tension and mystery that the Scriptures present. No one knew better than Jesus that God was providentially ordering the universe, and yet even He cried out with loud tears facing the way in front of Him.

My arrogance was shattered when a doctor told my wife and me that he didn't think my wife would ever be able to carry a child to term. I am ashamed to say that my response went from grief to submerged anger. I felt entitled to a "normal" life as I defined it—including the children I'd always assumed would be part of our lives. In His kindness, God used a visit from a friend to convict me of sin and lead me to a place of trust. This friend stopped by to visit us after the third of our miscarriages, right after the doctor had given us that devastating word. He was a respected historical theologian, one with a very high view of God's sovereignty. As a matter of fact, one of his books had convinced me, as a young seminarian, of just what the Bible teaches on God's providential direction of all things. I expected him to talk about remembering that God was in control. He didn't. He knew we were already convinced of that. What we needed was what he did. He cried with us, prayed with us, and, as he was walking out the door, said to me, "Russell I don't know why God is permitting this to happen to you right now, but I know this: Jesus is alive. He is present with you in your life right now." This man then pointed me to Psalm 27:4: "One thing have I asked of the LORD, that will I seek after: that I may dwell in the house of the LORD all the days of my life, to gaze upon the beauty of the LORD and to inquire in his temple." This older man said to me, "We will keep praying that the Lord will grant you children, but, even if He does not, He has already given to you the one thing you have asked of Him. He has given you life in Christ Jesus." That was what I needed to hear.

Now, many years later, our house is filled with clamor all around me, as five sons whirl about all over this house, even as I write this right now. The doctors, in our case, were wrong. We adopted two sons and then had three more the more typical way. Our story ended happily, but that happiness is not because God gave us children. Our story ends happily because God is for us—and has shown that to us in the sacrificial offering and triumphant resurrection of Jesus. We make all sorts of requests to Him, but, in truth, all of that amounts to just one thing: to dwell in the house of the Lord forever.

I thought about this hard lesson we learned many times as I read this beautiful book by Chelsea Patterson Sobolik. She, like us, walked through many dangers, toils, and snares—grappling with her longing for motherhood. You should read this book if you are in the same situation as she is in, as I was in, but you should read it even if you are not. There is someone around you right now who is hurting, with dreams deferred, or destroyed, of being a mother or a father. Maybe it's you or maybe it's someone who sits behind you at church. Chelsea bears witness here powerfully, because she does not attempt to "spin" her own reactions into something that will sound more spiritually admirable. She is honest about reacting with envy and anger when she sees the pregnant woman with two children in the grocery store ice-cream aisle. But she doesn't end with her hurt. She returns again and again to the gospel she clung to from the beginning. She returns to that one thing she asked of the Lord: "Remember me when you come into your kingdom" (Luke 23:42).

God answered Chelsea's prayers, and not just for her eternal good. He also answered her prayers for motherhood. No, she doesn't give us some prosperity-gospel manual for how to miraculously procreate despite the physical impossibility. Instead, she gives us something better. She shows us how the Scripture teaches us that mothering is not just a matter of biology. God has given Chelsea a calling to cultivate life, to mother children, and she is doing just that. The household of God, biblically defined, is more important than our familial households (as important as they are).

Maybe you picked up this book because you received a devastating diagnosis of infertility. Maybe you're reading this, afraid to go to the doctor, but growing more fearful as you see, month after month, that lonely one line on the pregnancy test instead of two. Maybe you're praying with loved ones who are longing to be parents and don't see it happening for them. This book is a book of good news. This book is a word of testimony that resonates with that of our ancestors in the faith, the three exiles in Babylon, who refused to bow down to the golden statue of Nebuchadnezzar the king. When told their sentence was to be burned alive, their response was simple. "If this be so, our God whom we serve is able to deliver us from the burning fiery furnace, and he will deliver us out of your hand, O king," they said. "But if not, be it known to you, O king, that we will not serve your gods or worship the golden image that you have set up" (Dan. 3:17–18). Those words "but if not" are crucial. They did not worship God because He gave them what they wanted. They worshipped God because He is God, and asked Him to answer their longings. If their worship was rendered only when they could see God's deliverance visibly, there would have been no issue with bowing to an idol because they would have already been doing so: to an idol of their imagination that they called "God." They were people, though not of idolatry but of faith.

Infertility can feel like a fiery furnace. It may even be worse, because a furnace would consume a person in a matter of minutes while the quiet agony of infertility can sometimes last for years. Chelsea stands here for us as one who has come through the furnace. And, like those in Babylon before her, there is no smell of fire on her (see Dan. 3:27). That's not because she doesn't suffer, but because God has not left her alone. I fully expect that sometime after this book is published and in your hands, Chelsea will, in fact, find herself a mother of children, just as her own mother did. "But if not," she is not deprived. She is a mother within the family of Christ—shaping and forming the generation to come. More importantly, she is crucified with Christ and is in Him raised from the dead and seated at the right hand of God forever.

Children are a blessing from the Lord. But childlessness does not mean loneliness. Chelsea shows us how. If you're longing to be a mother (or a father) or if you know someone who is, this book can help you. This book can teach you how to pray, how to bear each other's burdens, and how to find hope in what seems to be hopelessness. This book can point you toward joy, the joy of knowing that God has answered your deepest prayer, if you know Christ. You have no empty table. You are destined for a table bustling with brothers and sisters. In the meantime, pray and ask God for children, if you desire them. And while you're at it, be—like so many of our mothers in the faith—one who parents the church through the Word of God.

Along the way, though, remember what is so hard for all of us to remember: "One thing I have asked of you, to dwell in your house forever, to see your beauty forever."

Your prayers are answered. Everything else that God answers, and in whatever way He answers, those things, are just signposts to that.

RUSSELL MOORE

INTRODUCTION

*M*y adoptive parents had the privilege of meeting the teenage girl who brought me into the world. Over the years, they told me stories about her sitting in a cold apartment in Romania, holding me as tears fell down her cheeks and knowing that she'd never be able to be my mother . . . knowing that she was about to give up her daughter and—at least for that time in her life—her motherhood.

My story begins in that former communist nation in the capital city of Bucharest. Romania was under the rule of one of the cruelest dictators in Eastern Europe, Nicolae Ceaușescu. He held the beautiful country in a proverbial iron grip for almost a quarter of a century. Under his dictatorship, the people of Romania suffered greatly beneath the restrictions of rationed food, constant surveillance, and persecution and imprisonment.

In an effort to compete with the Soviet Union's population, Ceaușescu devised a plan to increase Romania's population from 23 million to 30 million by 2000. In 1966, he enacted a decree that essentially made pregnancy a state policy and proclaimed that the "fetus is the property of the entire society" and that anyone who avoided having children would be deemed "a deserter who abandons the laws of national continuity." Women under the age of forty-five were routinely brought in by authorities for check-ups, and if they hadn't become pregnant within a certain time frame, they'd be subject to a "celibacy tax."[1]

A result of this cruel policy—a consequence that lasted far beyond Ceauşescu's death by execution in 1989 —was that women were forced to have children they couldn't take care of, leaving half a million children as wards of the state. Parents abandoned their children by the droves, because they didn't have the financial or material resources to take care of them. The majority of children placed in communist orphanages weren't actual orphans; they were simply children whose parents were unable to care for them. Such orphanages were known as the "slaughterhouses of souls."[2]

Although I was spared such a place, I was one of those babies whose mother couldn't afford to keep her child. My birth mother was a nineteen-year-old girl with no money, no husband, and limited resources. Her decision to place me up for adoption wasn't an easy one. My birth mom longed for motherhood, but instead she had to *choose* childlessness.

Bobby and Christie Patterson were the two people God ordained to become my parents. They were in their late thirties and had lived a full life in the fifteen years they'd been married. Their love for adventure took them all over the world, including West Africa where they spent a year helping build a church.

When my parents got married in their early twenties, they didn't want children. In fact, they had made a deal before marrying that children wouldn't be a part of their life together. Within the first few years of their marriage, both of them came to know Christ as their personal Savior. As the Lord worked on their hearts, they discovered a desire to have children. But children didn't come. They walked through year after year of trying to conceive and explored different treatments that didn't seem to help. Finally, my mom conceived, but a few short months later, she miscarried. They were back to square one.

In 1990, right after my father had started his own architectural firm, my parents found their longing for parenthood intensifying, and they also found themselves in the middle of an excruciatingly long domestic adoption process. During that time, they had conversations with several couples who were also considering international adoption. Finding friends in a similar stage of life and walking toward the same goal made them feel like they weren't alone.

One night, a call came seemingly out of the blue from my dad's business partner who told him a *20/20* documentary called "Shame of a Nation" about the Romanian orphans was airing and that they should watch it. My dad almost dismissed it until my mom's sister called and suggested the very same thing. They decided to watch the documentary and invited their friends over to join them, not knowing that one hour would forever change their lives.

They learned that soon after Ceaușescu was executed in a revolution on Christmas Day in 1989, the Western world quickly arrived in Romania. What they found were thousands of children existing in horrible state-run institutions. The documentary introduced the world—and Bobby and Christie Patterson—to these children, struggling to survive. In the days following, my parents prayed about what they'd just witnessed. Starving children. Disabled children. Children who had experienced massive amounts of trauma. My parents asked themselves, "Is this our chance to become parents?" The Lord had begun to place a desire on their hearts to travel to Romania to adopt. Five weeks later, they were on a plane with their friends, bound for the adventure of a lifetime.

One of their deepest prayers while they were in Romania was that the Lord would intentionally guide them to the children He wanted them to adopt. It seemed like an almost impossible prayer. There were so many needy children; would the Lord *really* direct them to the ones He'd ordained for them? Through a series of events, several Romanians stepped up and began helping my parents with the adoption process. They visited several orphanages, but also had the chance to visit some birth mothers who were planning on placing their children in an institution.

Several times, my parents met various children but didn't sense a peace about adopting any of them. There were other American couples in Romania hoping to adopt, and the process seemed quicker and easier for them than for my parents. My mom recounts going back to the dingy, cold apartment where they were staying and crying out to the Lord, "Have You brought me all this way, only to leave me without a child? It's not fair!" Even in the midst of the pain of so many other mothers and children, my mother was overwhelmed by the pain of her own longing.

A few days later, the Holy Spirit directed Bobby and Christie to my birth mother Ana and to me. Before I was even handed to my parents, my mom said she knew that I was going to be her daughter. Immediately they began the necessary paperwork to legally adopt me. Since Romania had just recently broken free of its communist leader, the government was still accustomed to working on a bribery system. My parents quickly learned that if they wanted to leave the country anytime soon, they'd have to pay extra cash so it would take weeks instead of months to process paperwork. Finally, after five weeks, they purchased plane tickets home to North Carolina.

In addition to finding and adopting me, they also adopted a little boy, eleven days older than I was. Ana, tears streaming down her cheeks, came to hold me one last time and say goodbye before my parents boarded the plane and headed back to the United States.

My parents went on to adopt four more children. Because the adoption laws changed in Romania, and foreigners were no longer allowed to adopt Romanian children, my parents went to other countries, and over the years, adopted a boy and three more girls, making the Patterson family complete.

While the beginning of my story started off rocky in the world's eyes, my heavenly Father was quietly and tenderly preparing me for things to come. Little did anyone know that the baby girl adopted from Romania would one day learn that she could never have babies of her own.

But I've also been discovering that what, at first, may look like a legacy of childlessness, the God of hope means for good.

ONE

THE SILENT STRUGGLE
Why Childlessness Can Feel Lonely

When I was eighteen, I grew concerned because, unlike so many of my friends, I still hadn't graduated into "full womanhood"—I hadn't started my period. My mother was aware of the fact that my body hadn't reached full maturity yet, but she assured me that everything was probably fine, and we could give things a bit more time. As the months passed, my period never began, and we scheduled a routine physical, expecting to be told that I was just a late bloomer.

My OB/GYN was a kind woman who tried her best to calm my nerves. I'd never been to a gynecologist before and wasn't looking forward to the awkwardness that was surely going to accompany my visit. Growing up in a conservative Christian family, topics like the development of my body and sex in general weren't openly discussed often. My parents were probably trying to be extra cautious because they wanted to guard our hearts and minds from the sexually explicit culture that was the context of our teen years. But as I fell behind in normal physical development, the conversations with my mom became more upfront.

At the end of my appointment, the doctor scheduled more tests in the upcoming months. Despite the lack of an exact diagnosis, the doctor had delivered devastating news. She gently explained to me that there was a possibility I would never be able to have my own children. I could hardly believe what I was hearing. She didn't offer any more information than that, and I was too scared to press her for more.

But I didn't have time to dwell on the "possibility." A few days later, I was packing up everything I owned and heading to Virginia to start my freshman year at Liberty University. The majority of my time and attention was focused on attending classes, making friends, and learning how to navigate college life. The one thing I didn't unpack was any further thoughts about my condition.

Before I knew it, Thanksgiving break came, and I could no longer avoid my fears. The possibility of not having biological children was another doctor's visit away. The night before my appointment, I locked myself in my room, facing a big unknown. What would the next day bring? Would the doctor confirm my worst fear? How could I go on living if my nightmare became true?

I had grown up in a family of six children and had been surrounded by other children my entire life. During many summers, I worked in the children's ministry at my local church, where I learned how to better share the love of Jesus with kids. Babysitting was my first "real" job, and I volunteered at summer camps for elementary and middle schools. I have a natural love for children and had always wanted to be a mom one day. Sure, I was looking forward to going to college, starting a career, meeting someone, falling in love, and getting married. But I'd always anticipated the day when my husband and I would find out that I was pregnant, share the good news with our friends and family, and start planning and preparing for our little one to enter the world. This was the natural course of life I was expecting and longing for.

One of my deepest longings was to step into the role of motherhood, and there I sat alone in my room with the looming possibility of being unable to bear children. So many different questions stared me in the face. "Would I ever conceive a child? How would I handle life if I wasn't able to bear my own children?" But the one that weighed on my heart most in the quiet moments was "Will I ever be a mother?"

That question screamed inside my soul as I feebly attempted to prepare for the next day. Everything in me hoped that I'd find out that my body was normal and that I could move on with my life as planned. But I was aware of the possible outcome. I grabbed a pen and wrote out two pages of the most comforting Scripture verses I could find, mostly from the book of Psalms. As I sat there reading verse after verse aloud, tears streamed down my cheeks, and I prayed and begged God for a favorable diagnosis. I didn't think I could bear it if I found out that I couldn't have children. My faith didn't feel strong enough if God denied me what my heart so desperately longed for.

The last words I heard as I finally drifted off to sleep were from the song "Healer" by Hillsong United. The lyrics about trusting God in the worst storms comforted me as I tried to remind myself that I wasn't alone in those difficult moments.

The next morning, my mom and I pulled up to the Starbucks drive-thru to buy some liquid fuel for the "big day," and she asked how I was feeling.

"Well, I've prayed up the best I can," I answered. "I've filled my heart and mind with Scripture, and I've gotten a good night's sleep. Past that, I don't really know what else I can do. I'm just ready to get this over with."

She smiled at me as she handed me my cup of coffee. We drove to the doctor's office, and she tried to reassure me with the words, "It's going to be okay."

Everything in me wanted to scream, "You don't know that! Stop offering me useless words!" Her attempt at comforting me fell flat on my troubled heart.

As with many young women, my relationship with my mother was complicated during my teenage years. I was homeschooled from preschool through high school, and the closer college came, the more I wanted to break free, spread my wings, and fly away from home as fast as possible. My mother and I are very different. She's a no-nonsense woman who raised and homeschooled six children. The term "Mama Bear" accurately describes her, because everything she does is out of her fierce love for and loyalty to her children. A quality I most admire about her now—her ability to be blunt—used to drive me crazy. My response to pain is to withdraw, which made communicating during the early months of this trial even more difficult for the two of us. We had a tough time navigating how we gave and received care and comfort, and although she was the closest person to me, she's also the person I hurt the most.

Her motivation in the car that day was as pure as gold, but I was scared, and in that moment didn't appreciate overly simplistic attempts at support. But I couldn't blame her for her response; I hadn't shared with her the depth of my feelings and doubts. A part of me felt scared to verbalize all the fears that lurked in my mind. If I kept them to myself, maybe they wouldn't come to be. While I wanted to lash out at her seeming lack of understanding, I couldn't possibly understand everything going on in my own heart. So I only nodded to acknowledge her words, and we finished the drive to the doctor in silence.

As we got out of the car, the chilly autumn air hit my skin, and I gripped my coffee cup tighter to warm up. We walked into the lobby and were handed a stack of paperwork to fill out. I was thankful for the distraction while I was waiting to be called back. Each moment that passed felt like an eternity. Finally, my name was called, and I was greeted by overly enthusiastic nurses who instructed me to slip into a hospital gown. I was guided to the MRI machine and lay there silent and still, but my mind was racing. I felt something wet on my face. Completely unaware that I had been crying, I realized that I had never felt more alone in my life. As much as my family wanted to support me, no one could physically take my place that day. The same questions that flooded my mind the night before were back and even more overwhelming than before.

Later, as I waited in the examination room for the

doctor to come and explain the results to me, all I could think to do was to silently beg the Lord to be with me. At last the doctor arrived, I could tell from the moment she walked in that she didn't have good news to share. Her facial expression was solemn, and although her voice was quiet, her words hit my heart like a sledgehammer: "Sweetheart, you were born with a rare condition that has left you without a uterus." Before I had time to begin processing this, she jumped into explaining what this meant for my future. "You won't ever be able to carry your own child."

I looked at her stunned. I fought for breath to fill my lungs, and in one breath from the doctor, my life was forever changed. I had been born with Mayer-Rokitansky-Küster-Hauser (MRKH) syndrome, a rare condition with a 100 percent guarantee that I'd never be able to carry my own children. When my body was being formed in my mother's womb, some reproductive organs failed to form. There I was at nineteen years old—the same age Ana was when she placed me for adoption—realizing that, biologically, I could never be a mother. As I tried wrapping my mind around this news, I left the appointment and was back in the car with my mom. I was too shocked to cry; all I felt was numbness. It took a few days for the shock to turn into myriad emotions—sadness, frustration grief, shame, anger, and loneliness.

Ironically, Thanksgiving Day was a few days after the appointment, and the last thing in my heart was thankfulness. Instead of counting my blessings, all I could focus on were the losses in my body. Life already seemed to be moving on without me. Family arrived at our house that Thursday to gather around the table, eat a giant meal, and enjoy the holiday together. All I wanted to do was escape to my room and be by myself. No one but my parents knew about my diagnosis at this point, and I was ashamed to tell everyone else. I was worried that they'd immediately see me in a different light, and all that would define me was my inability to have children. So, I mustered up all the courage I could, dried my tears, and spent the day with the family.

After the Thanksgiving break, I headed back to college, a completely different woman than when I'd left. The news that I would be childless sent me into an emotional tailspin. It was too much to bear alone, but I was ashamed to tell people, so I withdrew from friends and family. For the first few weeks, I was able to stuff all my emotion and grief inside me and make it through the day. I'd rush back to my dorm room just in time to have a breakdown but was able to keep it hidden from people. That is, until I experienced my first panic attack.

It was a chilly winter day as I headed out to enjoy our college team play basketball. I met up with a group of my friends and tried to focus on having a good time, but the familiar ache of sadness was still on my heart. All of a sudden, I couldn't catch my breath, and I felt like walls were closing in on me. I'd just experienced the first of many panic attacks. The anxiety I'd been carrying in my heart forced its way out. A panic attack is a "sudden episode of intense fear that triggers severe physical reactions."[1] I was so afraid of not being loved or supported. In addition to my anxiety and sadness, I struggled with loneliness. All my emotions seemed to force themselves out in panic attacks.

As I continued to process my diagnosis, my mind was assaulted by self-doubt and lies from the enemy. I felt as if

I wasn't a whole woman. If my body couldn't even fulfill the basic physical functions of a woman, what good was I? Would any man ever want me if I couldn't provide him with children? The Christian culture I was immersed in seemed to promote the idea that a woman's highest calling was to be a mother, and my heart longed for motherhood. If I couldn't fulfill this expected role, was I somehow receiving God's punishment?

Despite the earliest days of my childhood, childlessness was my first real encounter with personal suffering. Until that point, my life had been comfortable and easy. I found myself forced to wrestle with my faith like never before and came to a spiritual fork in the road. I had no framework for suffering, and childlessness is an intense trial that affects you and those who love you forever. I found myself in the fight of a lifetime—a fight to hold on to my faith. Chances are, if you're reading this book, you're all too familiar with this grueling battle. I wish I could tell you that my immediate response to my suffering was to trust the Lord and to rest in His love. But I didn't.

Instead, I found myself struggling with frequent panic attacks, depression, and feeling traumatized in public places, because there were constant reminders of what I was lacking. Even a trip to the grocery store could be a struggle. Once, I was standing in the frozen food section of Walmart, trying to decide which ice cream flavor I wanted. I saw a mom with two young children who were jumping all over the place, obviously excited about buying ice cream. I tried not to look in their direction, but they came closer and closer to me. Surely, they didn't want mint chocolate chip too!

"Get away from me," I thought. "There are a million

other flavors, and I don't want children near me right now." I turned to the family to give them a look of annoyance, only to notice that the mother was pregnant. That was the last straw, and I stood there crying in the ice cream aisle. This scene wasn't an isolated event but one that played itself out dozens of times over the years.

Because the pain could be unpredictable, emotion would grip my heart at the most inconvenient times. But how God chose to show His care for me could be just as surprising. One day in class, as my professor droned on and on about political philosophy, my mind drifted off to my grief. It didn't take long for the tears to come, and I hurried to the nearest bathroom, sobbing. The custodian walked in on me having a meltdown, but instead of ignoring me or walking out, she came and sat on the bench beside me, put her arm around me, and held me until I calmed down. I shared with her what caused my breakdown, and she knelt on the bathroom floor and prayed over me.

Unlike my personal times of prayer, which were lately characterized by wondering if following Jesus was worth the heartache I felt like He had caused, this precious woman's prayer was refreshing, as was the fact that she knew about my childlessness and lifted me up in prayer. I was trying to reconcile my childlessness with my professed beliefs about God's goodness and sovereignty, and she was lending me her faith when mine was weak. Throughout my time at college, this woman always made it a point to ask how I was doing every time she saw me. God was quietly showing me His care, too, even in the most unlikely places.

By God's grace, I'm still a Christian in spite of walking

through this horrible experience. I've wrestled with the Lord, screamed my pain, and groaned my prayers. Nevertheless, He's kept me. I resolved before the Lord that I would follow Him no matter the cost. Throughout this book, we'll look at ways to mourn childlessness. The cost might feel too great at times, but I promise that the Lord will hold you fast on this journey.

A FAMILIAR JOURNEY

This may be surprising, but childlessness touches the lives of many women, and the precious people who love them. Infertility alone affects approximately 12 percent of the US population—that's over one in ten couples![2] According to estimates, roughly 15 to 20 percent of all pregnancies in the US will end in miscarriage.[3] The risk of miscarriage in known pregnancies under twelve weeks is one in five.[4]

Despite these numbers, the data doesn't encompass couples who have lost children to illness or accidents, nor does it take into consideration single women who desire to be mothers. Those nearing the end of the ideal childbearing years with no prospects for marriage on the horizon often desire to be mothers, but their singleness has other plans.

Whatever your personal experience with childlessness, the first thing to hold on to is that you're not alone, even when you feel like you are. Because it can be difficult to share your particular journey with childlessness, it's helpful to remember that there are many women experiencing the same trial—often experiencing it in silence.

In addition, infertility, barrenness, and miscarriage are still taboo subjects, especially in the Christian culture.

Probably without realizing it, churches may isolate the childless by not integrating the subject into the regular conversations of the life of the church.

If so many people struggle with being childless, why isn't this a conversation that's had more often? I believe one of the reasons is that the church often doesn't know how to respond appropriately to pain. People's hearts are often in a good place and desiring to help, but they simply don't know how. One of the first steps to creating safe places is by raising awareness. When pastors and their flocks are more conscious of the childless in their midst, they'll begin changing their language, what they joke about, and the questions they ask.

Often there aren't enough safe places, even in our churches, for us to come together to share our stories, our longings, and our losses. In my own experience, I have been shocked that there aren't more books, more support groups, and more willingness to be open on this topic. When I was fighting to hang on, fighting to hold on to my faith, I felt like no one understood what I was going through. The lack of available resources propelled my desire to write this book.

The book you hold in your hands is a labor of love. I feel like I've written it in blood instead of ink. Dear reader, I've prayed over you with such intensity. While I don't know you by name, the Lord does. The world may never know how many tears you've cried, but you can rest in the fact that not one tear has fallen to the ground without God noticing. Are you ready to begin this messy journey together? I can't promise that it'll be easy. In fact, there will be moments when you may feel like giving up. But I can promise that if you keep moving forward, by God's grace you'll begin to find the healing you so desperately long for. As I type these words, my physical circumstances haven't changed, although I am engaged and will soon marry Michael, the love of my life. I haven't seen the Lord redeem my trial as I would have liked. I'm not on the other side of it, holding a beautiful baby, happy and satisfied. If I'm honest, there are still nights when I cry myself to sleep, days when I wrestle with the Lord because I can't have a child. I'm still in the middle of this journey, right beside you in your childlessness.

Childlessness is a heartbreaking experience, and my desire is that those experiencing it will begin to feel more comfortable sharing their trial with their communities of faith, family, and friends.

SHAME KEEPS US SILENT

Many women feel shame mingled with their sorrow. It is easy to believe that you don't have children because of something you have done or failed to do. People are quick to offer their (frequently unhelpful) opinions and advice when you're experiencing a trial, particularly one as intimate as childlessness. As Karen Rivers, director of the Solace Foundation, a nonprofit organization that offers comfort and support to parents after the loss of a pregnancy or infant, says about miscarriage, "The isolation is huge. It's not something that's talked about, because it makes people uncomfortable, and it makes people sad. My hope is that we're getting better in terms of awareness, but I think it's still largely taboo."[5]

Even though I have experienced only one of the forms that childlessness can take, I'm well acquainted with the grief of being unable to have a child. This heartache has forever stained my heart with sorrow. The desire for children is often one of the most intense longings you can feel. Not only are you struggling with an unfulfilled desire, but a private and often unspoken struggle. No one knows that you can't have children or are struggling unless you tell them. No one knows the sorrow of your heart or how heavy and difficult this situation can be. Childlessness is not a visible pain. It's not easily on display for the world to see. When someone walks through a visible trial, such as an illness, while still difficult, the fact that it's unconcealed makes the way clearer for talking to others.

Despite the fact that we live in a society with increasing access to information and to social networks, childlessness remains a taboo topic that many people aren't comfortable discussing. As a result, this topic doesn't receive the attention it needs, especially from Christians. Because we don't always experience a culture of openness, a woman might not feel safe being the first one to begin the process of sharing.

CHILDLESSNESS AFFECTS EVERY PART OF A PERSON

The struggle toward motherhood can affect every part of your life. Research from Harvard Medical School has shown that women with infertility have the same levels of anxiety and depression as do women with cancer and heart disease. The same study reveals that many women who experience childlessness say that it's the most upsetting experience of their lives.[6] For some, childlessness may be their first major encounter with suffering and can quickly lead to their faith being tested and tried in the furnace. When I first began walking through childlessness, I wanted everyone I came into contact with to know how deeply I was hurting. I wanted to wear my hurt and my heart on my sleeve. I longed for empathy and encouragement. Even though my childlessness was an intimate detail about me, and I didn't necessarily want everyone to know *why* I was suffering, I still wanted people to know that I was hurting. My soul longed to be seen and loved, but I felt like I was in a cocoon of my own emotions.

If you're walking through childlessness, chances are you feel as if your heart is breaking and the suffering is agonizing. Did you know that having a broken heart is a scientifically proven phenomenon? It's called "Broken Heart Syndrome," and women are more likely than men to experience the intense chest pain, a reaction to the surge of stress hormones that can be caused by an emotionally stressful event. This pain, accompanied by shortness of breath can almost feel like a heart attack.[7] I experienced frequent panic attacks as I began processing my barrenness. The pain that's deep inside your heart demands to make its way out. If you're experiencing physical pain of this nature, recognize that the link between your mind, heart, and body is strong. These types of physical manifestations are common when going through something this difficult.

Suffering is hard. Suffering alone is almost unbearable. One of the things that makes childlessness so difficult is the fact that it's such an intimate experience. A woman's fertility, or lack thereof, is typically viewed as an integral part of her identity. When her ability to reproduce is compromised, it can cause immense shame on top of sadness. Childlessness can even be humiliating, because it contradicts what we know about the created order of the world. God created us to be nurturers. Although not every woman longs for motherhood, it is a godly desire. Our physical composition tells of this truth. We have breasts to feed a newborn; we have a uterus to grow a fetus. Our bodies were intentionally designed to fulfill God's mandate to "be fruitful and multiply." However, the fall continues to taint everything in our imperfect world. Things aren't the way they should be—they aren't the way God originally designed them to be.

ACKNOWLEDGING EXTERNAL PRESSURES

While our longing for motherhood is normal and natural, oftentimes it's intensified by external pressures. Well-meaning family members can often place a huge burden on the shoulders of their loved ones. Asking one too many times when they'll start their own family or give them grandbabies can be devastating for the couple who is struggling.

Some of the greatest pressure to be a mother can actually come from within the church. Christians have a tendency to take good things and fashion them into the ultimate goal. Hence the elevation of motherhood into the ultimate goal of womanhood. Oh, how this breaks my heart! Being a woman is so much more than being a wife and mother. When the church elevates motherhood to a place that it shouldn't be, it is unintentionally implying that once you've become a mother, you'll be more satisfied, more fulfilled, more of a woman than before. Women who don't have (or can't have) children may feel alienated, humiliated, and afraid to vocalize their struggle. I've attended far too many churches where single women, or married women without children, simply don't fit in well because the church culture doesn't make room for them. Small groups are a way in which this issue often plays out in local churches. Far too often, small groups are created based on age or life stage. Women who are of childbearing age are often lumped into groups with young mothers. These types of well-meaning groups can easily stir up jealousy and pain in the hearts of childless women.

While being a wife and a mother are both noble goals and callings, they don't have to be our primary goals as women. Motherhood has its own unique challenges for stay-at-home mothers, single mothers, working moms, etc. The church often doesn't dwell on the difficulties of motherhood. Instead they tend to gloss over the hardships and paint motherhood to be the most desirable role possible.

We know from Scripture that we can learn to be content in any and every circumstance, but when we're walking through one of the most difficult trials a woman may face, the pain can be intensified when the church is unintentionally insensitive.

In a later chapter, I'll discuss this further and suggest ways that churches and pastors can begin changing this culture, in order to love well those who are experiencing childlessness. For now, it's enough to acknowledge that the church can be one of the loneliest places for those of us walking through this particular struggle.

FIERCE FEMININITY

Femininity and womanhood are so much grander and more beautiful than we're often taught. Women are created in the image of our Creator. God intentionally and carefully designed us. The greatest role of a woman is not to be a mother, but rather, to glorify God with our whole lives in whatever circumstances we find ourselves. Biblical womanhood is about boldness, tenacity, tender heartedness, and loving the Lord and His people. As Elisabeth Elliot wrote:

> To understand the meaning of womanhood we have to start with God. If He is indeed "Creator of all things visible and invisible" He is certainly in charge of all things, visible and invisible, stupendous and minuscule, magnificent and trivial. God has to be in charge of details if He is going to be in charge of the overall design.[8]

The Hebrew word used in Genesis to describe Eve, the very first woman, is *ezer*. This term means "help" and is used to denote strength or power. It occurs twenty-one times in the Old Testament. In many of the Psalms, *ezer* is used to describe God's character and the way He interacts with His people. Here are a few examples:

Psalm 20:2—May he send you *help* from the sanctuary and give you support from Zion!

Psalm 33:20—Our soul waits for the Lord; he is our *help* and our shield.

Psalm 115:9—O Israel, trust in the Lord! He is their *help* and their shield.

Psalm 121:1–2—I lift my eyes to the hills. From where does my *help* come? My *help* comes from the LORD, who made heaven and earth.

WOMEN AS THE WEAKER SEX?

Women are generally more nurturing than men. The way God designed us can often cause society to view us as the weaker sex. In our feminist-leaning society, we take insult with the label "weaker sex." We demand to be treated just as equally as men, and we bristle when we hear the church talk about us as "helpmates." However, the identity God gave us isn't "lesser than" a man's identity at all. We're created differently, and that's a good thing. Men and women complement one another in ways that reflect the Trinity.

In fact, the power the Lord has placed in our hearts is fiery and fierce. Women are not only warriors, we're also a fortress. We were created to be a safe place, a shield, a help, and a comfort. When we're modeling these characteristics to the world, we're saying something about God. These characteristics manifest themselves even in our bodies—yes, during pregnancy but also in the marriage relationship. In the most physically intimate act between a husband and a wife, the woman's body is designed to be a safe place, literally a shield for the man in his most physically vulnerable state.

God crafted a woman's body and spirit to reflect Him in such a powerful way. So often, we can feel ashamed or annoyed that we're referred to as a "helper," but if we read it in its original biblical context, it's one of the greatest honors God could have given to women.

In 1 Peter 3:4, women are instructed to "let your adorning be the hidden person of the heart with the imperishable beauty of a gentle and quiet spirit, which in God's sight is very precious." In their book *True Beauty*, Carolyn Mahaney and Nicole Whitacre explain that "a gentle and quiet spirit is not a personality trait. It is the quality of a woman who meets adversity—slander, sickness, rejection, and loss—with a calm confidence."[9]

When I found out I couldn't have children, that my body was made differently than most women, that I was a woman without a womb, I began to question my usefulness and even my existence on this earth. I thought, "If I can't even fulfill the basic duties of a woman, what good am I?"

Have you had similar thoughts? Have you felt like your worth is tied to your ability to have children? Be assured that your value isn't dependent on your ability to conceive or bear babies. I realize those words are easy to say, but much harder to actually believe.

For years, one of my biggest fears—and a self-imposed pressure—was that I wouldn't be loved by a man because I can't have children. I was afraid that if I were fully known, I would never be fully loved because of this huge secret I'd kept for so long. I feared I would be rejected and remain unloved based on the defects of my body. Thankfully, these fears haven't come to pass, but these are lies I'm regularly tempted to believe. We must constantly remind ourselves that a woman is no less feminine if she's unmarried, without children, or unable to carry children. Our womanhood is based on who God says we are—and nothing less.

GRIEVING IN THE MIDST OF THE SILENCE

When I began baring my soul to close friends and sharing about my childlessness, many people's first reactions were, "Oh, Chelsea, I'm so sorry. But it'll all be okay—

you can just adopt children." What those precious friends weren't getting was the fact that I was sharing something incredibly intimate about myself, this information was breaking my heart, and I needed them to grieve with me. I needed someone to be there with me to say, "I don't really know what to do or say right now, but I'm right here, grieving with you, ready to love and care for you in whatever ways you need."

Our general response to pain is typically one of two things—either we're fearful of the pain and want to run away from it or eliminate it as quickly as possible, or our pain becomes the most important thing in our lives. With the private trial of childlessness, more often than not, we try to minimize our pain. Because of the private nature of our struggle, we may often find that people don't know how to comfort us. They might be scared that they won't offer the right words of comfort, or that they'll be too intrusive, so they remain silent. Both sides can struggle to know how to approach this trial well. As a result, we can be scared to quiet our hearts and feel the reality of the situation. It's uncomfortable; it hurts.

Too often, we rush through pain, because we want to get to the other side. We want to feel "okay again." We want to return to a normal life. We don't like to sit with the pain, because there's an uncertainty and unpredictability to suffering. You never know what your heart will and won't be able to bear. But don't be afraid of tears; don't be afraid to truly mourn and to feel the hurt. It's completely normal to grieve an unfulfilled desire. Because if you're experiencing childlessness—either for a season or indefinitely—you're essentially mourning the death of what could have been. You're mourning the death of a dream and in order to find healing and recapture hope, you must allow yourself to grieve.

When we're in pain, the last thing we need is for someone to attempt to fix it for us. Well-meaning friends often end up hurting our hearts more with responses that feel like salt in a wound. And when we're not given the freedom to grieve, we begin to keep our emotions to ourselves, instead of sharing. We don't know who in our community we can really trust with our heart and our sorrow. David wept, Job wept, Hannah wept, even Jesus wept. Why aren't we allowed to weep and lament without someone rushing in, slapping a few Bible verses on our problems, and expecting us to "get over it" and be okay? As singer-songwriter Michael Card wrote in his book on suffering titled *A Sacred Sorrow*, "It seems to me that we do not need to be taught how to lament. What we need is simply the assurance that we can lament."[10]

One of the biggest ways the Western church can grow is to learn that sorrow, grief, and lament aren't things to run away from. Life is a painful journey toward heaven, and Christians should learn how to have tender hearts. The grief of another is an opportunity for the church to put Galatians 6:2 into practice as we "bear one another's burdens."

CHANGING YOUR PERSONAL PERSPECTIVE

It's important that we feel free to share our trial with family, friends, and our local church communities. And as we begin journeying toward hope together, I want to remind you that God promises never to leave or forsake us. Even though our feelings might tell us otherwise, we can stake our hope on the fact that He'll be with us every step of the way. He sees you, knows you, and loves you.

There's no doubt that this trial is going to change you. When you've walked through childlessness—whether for a season or a lifetime—your heart will never be the same. My greatest prayer as we begin this journey deeper into grief and toward hope and healing is that you know Christ. Right now, as your heart is breaking, you might not feel close to Him, but I can guarantee that He's right beside you because He promises to be close to the brokenhearted.

I urge you to read this book through the lens of God's goodness, sovereignty, and great love for you. I can't answer all your questions; I can't tell you why the Lord allowed you to walk through this particular trial. But I can identify with your pain, I know the sorrow your heart has been through, and I can offer to walk the road toward hope alongside you.

Oh, may Christ be enough for us, even in the midst of childlessness! In great suffering on earth, there is great support from heaven. Four of the sweetest words ever spoken by God are, "I am with you."

> Be strong and courageous. Do not fear or be in dread of them, for it is the LORD your God who goes with you. He will not leave you or forsake you. (Deut. 31:6)

Our Father has promised never to leave us, never to forsake us, always to love us, and to work all things together for our ultimate good. Much of the time we don't understand why He's doing something, but we have a choice to make. We can choose to trust Him or to run away from Him. Even though we don't understand, we can choose to trust that our Father is with us . . .

When our heart is torn into pieces.

When the Lord hasn't answered our questions.

When we don't know if everything will be okay.

When the Lord hasn't promised to work in the ways that we want.

When the pain threatens to overshadow our vision of the Lord.

And I encourage you to hold on to the Lord's promises to us in Scripture:

He promises to be present (Matt. 28:20).

He promises us His love (Rom. 5:8).

He promises us His grace (Ps. 86:15).

He promises to sustain us (Ps. 55:22).

He promises us His aid (Heb. 13:6).

He promises steadfastness (Ps. 31:7).

He promises provision (Phil. 4:19).

I'm so happy you are taking steps toward hope and healing. Wherever you're at on this journey, recognize that it's okay to not be okay. It's okay to limp, it's okay to fall, it's okay to be quiet, and it's okay to wail out your pain. God is big enough to handle it. Being seen and loved in the midst of this trial will make all the difference in the world. May this not remain a silent struggle for you anymore.

REFLECTION & DISCUSSION

How have you responded to childlessness (e.g., anger, frustration, fear, sadness, guilt)? Spend time writing out the types of emotions that surround this trial.

Do you feel alone in your suffering? If so, what's making you feel like you can't share (e.g., shame, lack of support, fear)?

What are some external factors that make you feel pressured to be a mother?

Think about three trustworthy people with whom you can share your experience of childlessness.

Which promise of God listed at the end of the chapter stands out and why? Spend some time memorizing a few verses!

How do you see God's grace and love in this chapter?

_____

_____

_____

_____

_____

_____

_____

_____

_____

_____

_____

_____

_____

_____

_____

_____

_____

_____

_____

_____

_____

_____

_____

_____

_____

_____

_____

_____

TWO

SEASONS OF SORROW

What Do You Do in the Midst of Sorrow?

Sorrow interrupts our world like nothing else does. It barges in uninvited and reorients our hearts and lives. When we encounter deep trials, we know that we will never be the same, and life as we knew it is forever altered. As we journey through childlessness, we'll have to go to deep and dark places before we reach the light. This isn't an easy path. But I pray that on this journey, your heart can feel the freedom to grieve. Brokenness can be the starting point for healing. Without first recognizing where we actually are, we'll be unable to move past it and on to better and more beautiful things.

One moment, one sentence, has the power to change

your entire life. My life-changing moment arrived in the doctor's office when I was informed that I was biologically unable to bear children. In a few short minutes, I learned that I was a woman without a womb. Think about your own turning point. Was it the time you eagerly took a pregnancy test only to realize that it was negative again? Was it the first (or fifth) time a well-meaning person at church asked when you were going to get married so you could "get started with your life" and become a mother? Was it the time you went in for an ultrasound and the doctor couldn't find the heartbeat?

Each one of us has probably had experiences that changed everything. For some, perhaps it was a slower accumulation of many quieter moments: another negative pregnancy test, another trip through Target avoiding the baby section, another phone call from a friend declined because the conversation would be too painful. For others, that change was instant and traumatic: a miscarriage, a baby delivered stillborn, the unexpected death of a child. Chances are this book has triggered memories like this and the familiar ache in your heart for motherhood.

When I found out that I couldn't have children, my world stopped, and I was unwillingly thrown into the most difficult season I've ever walked through. The first few months were awful, and I cried more tears than I ever had. Everything I believed about God, His goodness, and His care for me was immediately brought into question. I began to ask God:

Why?
Why me?

If You really loved me, why would You do this?
What good could possibly come out of this?
Have I sinned in some way to deserve this?
Don't You know that I've tried to serve and obey You?
Why aren't You honoring that?

I imagine you've felt similar emotions and asked some of the same questions. Questioning the Lord feels like one of the most natural responses we can have in the midst of our pain. We have an aversion to pain and do our best to avoid it. However, avoidance isn't possible, and we must, at some point, face it. Oftentimes, questioning God is our first response. We want answers; we want to know the reasons behind the heartbreak. If we look through the psalms, we find the authors questioning the Lord. In one of the most gut-wrenchingly honest psalms from the pen of David, we find him hounding God for answers: "How long, O Lord? Will you forget me forever? How long will you hide your face from me? How long must I take counsel in my soul and have sorrow in my heart all the day? How long shall my enemy be exalted over me?" (Ps. 13:1–2).

As the days turned into months, my season of sorrow included depression, frequent panic attacks, withdrawing from friends and family—all while trying to understand God in the midst of this horrible heartache. For the first time in my life, my questions weren't being quickly answered, and I was angry about it. Frequently I found myself driving to a nearby warehouse parking lot in the evening, stopping under a streetlight, and crying. It was so helpful to have a place away from people where I could break down and cry, where I could scream my questions to the Lord, and where I could wail and mourn. Suffering isn't pretty. I don't think a genuine smile crossed my lips for months after I found out. I felt as if my identity and future had been snatched away from me, and I entered into a time of lament.

After Thanksgiving, I returned to college with this big secret in my soul. I was different than my peers and was silently mourning and trying to cope with my loss. My mother desperately tried to be there for me emotionally, but I pushed her away. Whenever I was upset, she would remind me that the Lord still loved me and that everything would ultimately be okay. That's *not* what I wanted to hear. Her blunt reminders of God weren't received well. I wanted someone to be angry at and lashed out at those closest to me. I was hurting, and in the moment, it felt good to hurt someone else.

For my mom and me, the trial of my childlessness changed us in a way I'm not sure anything else could have. By being thrown into the fire, we'd seen what we were made of. We discovered what we were lacking in our character. As I began to wrestle and grieve, my mother was quick to jump in with tales of her childlessness to try to comfort me by letting me know that she'd felt a similar pain. Her motivation was as pure as gold; however, I was offended every time she tried to do this because I was thinking, "Yes, but you were married when you went through childlessness. I'm unmarried, and *because* of my childlessness, I don't know if I'll ever find a man who'll want me."

Her attempt at comfort left me feeling even worse about myself. I felt so alone in my suffering and frustrated that the limited amount of comfort I was receiving wasn't helping. I took out my anger on my mother and spoke hurtful words. Grief can make us do things we're not proud of and that we wish we could take back. Praise God there's forgiveness in those intense times in the fire where we can so quickly lose control of ourselves.

In many ways, I viewed my mom as God's representative. As a loving and authoritative parental figure, she was the closest reflection of God, and because I felt like she was failing me, I also felt like God was failing me. I felt like God had abandoned me, wasn't listening to me, didn't understand me, or wasn't going to help me. Of course, I had all the head knowledge to tell me the opposite, but head knowledge can only get you so far. The road from the head to the heart is the longest road in the world.

In the months after my diagnosis, I began to carefully craft my days so I would avoid any interaction with children or pregnant women, even if that meant avoiding public places. Each of us has a different response to pain. While some of us might self-medicate with food, too much TV or social media, or excessive shopping, others of us turn inward, grit our teeth, and resolve to fight through the pain on our own. Still others might try to continually course correct and strive for perfection in hopes that our own goodness will bring us the blessing we so desperately desire. These are all normal and natural responses to stress, sorrow, and grief. Don't beat yourself up if you find yourself trying any of these coping strategies. Though I've tried them all at various times, I most often try to avoid pain by relying on my own work and effort to bring about divine purposes.

Growing up, I was always the "good girl," and I could usually rely on my actions to get what I wanted. If I was good enough, I'd receive a reward for my good behavior. My successes and failures seemed to rest on me and my actions. Now for the first time in my life, my "goodness" wasn't getting me a blessing. I easily began to view my relationship with the Lord in the same way. If I just worked hard enough, if I was good enough, or had enough faith, surely the Lord would bless me and give me what I wanted. But I found myself facing reality. I was born without a uterus—no amount of prayer could magically give me one. I knew that I was never going to bear children, and I couldn't understand why the Lord would let this happen.

Even though time has passed since that life-changing day, my heart still grieves what could have been. Time has a way of softening pain, so it doesn't feel quite as sharp or as constant, but the sorrow never completely leaves. Some women do eventually have their desired children and forget almost entirely the infertility or barrenness they once experienced. As it says in Proverbs, "A desire fulfilled is a tree of life" (Prov. 13:12). But all deep sorrow leaves a mark. Women who have experienced a miscarriage often say that their other children don't erase the pain of losing a baby. The child (or children) they never knew will forever remain in their hearts. Women who remain childless forever, either due to singleness or lifelong barrenness, will always feel the ache, though it may grow fainter with time.

By God's grace, my heart has experienced healing, but in order to be healed we must give ourselves time and space to be upset, to be angry, to weep, to mourn. Healing has been a long process for me. In a later chapter, I'll share more of that journey and how you can begin to heal. As much as I wish my healing looked like a straight line, it doesn't. I've been all over the place as I've healed and often feel like I take one step forward and two steps back! As you walk through childlessness, your heart is going to go through different stages of sorrow and grief as you begin to figure out how to adjust to a new reality. Whether temporary or permanent, childlessness comes with uncertainty, and there's no guarantee of a favorable outcome.

When I began chatting with other women I knew about childlessness, one of the most common threads in their stories was that they needed the space to feel and express raw and honest emotions. Katie and her husband, Javan, have been dear friends of mine for a few years. We've enjoyed leisurely dinners and chatting about life, love, and our relationship with the Lord. They have modeled an honest relationship with the Lord over the years, especially as they walked through three long years of infertility before finally finding that they were pregnant with their son. He made his appearance into the world almost three months early and spent excruciating days in the Neonatal Intensive Care Unit (NICU). The doctors and the nurses were fighting to keep breath flowing through his tiny body to keep him alive.

Katie confessed to me, "This wasn't how it was supposed to be. The long-awaited child wasn't supposed to come into the world like this. Will he be taken away from us too?" During the fight to keep their little boy alive, Katie and Javan would send out daily updates. Most of the updates were filled with questions they were wrestling with, prayer requests, and a plea for support from friends and family. What stood out to me about their journey is the fact that they weren't shy about expressing their hearts, even if they were messy. Their precious little one eventually got to go home, and I've been able to visit him since then. I hope his parents are able to share with him one day how the Lord worked in their lives during that time.

Every story of childlessness is unique in the details, but the heartbreak endured by the women and men walking this road is universal. The trial of childlessness changes you; you'll never be the same. Your world looks different because something you deeply long for has not come to pass. Despite your best efforts and without your approval, you're smack dab in the middle of a difficult and painful experience. Perhaps this is your first encounter with reality not matching up with your expectations, or maybe this feels like yet another thing that's stolen the breath from your lungs.

I can't remove the grief and sorrow from your heart, but I can provide some words of comfort to sustain you in the storm.

There are several strongholds I have clung to in the midst of my trial:

Cling to God's Promises

I've already touched on some of the promises of God in chapter 1, but grasping these has been the single most important thing I've done in walking through suffering. Write them down. Ask close friends to remind you of them. Do whatever it takes to fill your mind and heart with them.

The most helpful way I've found to remind myself of these truths is by memorizing Scripture verses that tell me who God is and what He'll do for me. Write down some of the verses you want to memorize on note cards and keep them close at all times. (I use spiral bound note cards.) What has helped me memorize Scripture is redeeming the "dead" time in my day. When I'm doing mindless tasks, I can be more intentional about filling my mind and heart with the Word of God. As I'm getting ready for work in the morning (blow drying my hair and doing my makeup), I either listen to my Bible app or have one of my Scripture note cards by my side to review. During my thirty-minute commute to work on public transportation, I focus my attention on feeding my soul.

It's always a good practice to hide God's Word in your heart, so when you encounter a particularly difficult situation, you'll already be armed with truth and be able to quickly recall God's promises. I encourage you to find these spaces in your schedule and be intentional about memorizing Scripture. Corrie ten Boom is credited with saying, "Gather the riches of God's promises. Nobody can take away from you those texts from the Bible which you have learned by heart."[1]

Some of my favorite Scriptures about God's promises are:

> I love you, O LORD, my strength. The LORD is my rock and my fortress and my deliverer, my God, my rock, in whom I take refuge, my shield, and the horn of my salvation, my stronghold. (Ps. 18:1–2)

> The LORD is a stronghold for the oppressed, a stronghold in times of trouble. And those who know your name put their trust in you, for you, O LORD, have not forsaken those who seek you. (Ps. 9:9–10)

You are a hiding place for me; you preserve me
from trouble; you surround me with shouts of
deliverance.... I will instruct you and teach you
in the way you should go; I will counsel you with
my eye upon you.... (Ps. 32:7–8)

The LORD is near to the brokenhearted and saves
the crushed in spirit. (Ps. 34:18)

Our soul waits for the LORD; he is our help and
our shield. For our heart is glad in him, because
we trust in his holy name. Let your steadfast love,
O LORD, be upon us, even as we hope in you.
(Ps. 33:20–22)

Say "Breath" Prayers

Stick with me on this one, because it might be a foreign
concept to you. A "breath" prayer is exactly what it
sounds like: a prayer you can pray in one breath. I've
found these to be so helpful when I'm exhausted and
don't have the energy to pray a long prayer. Since they can
be repeated over and over, they help to focus your mind
on truth. A few breath prayers I've prayed are as follows:

Lord, have mercy.
Not my will, but Yours be done.
My help comes from the Lord.
Show me Your glory.
When I'm afraid, I will trust in You.

Read Books about Suffering

In the early years of this journey, I devoured almost
every book I could find on the topic of suffering, since I

couldn't find a book on the topic of childlessness. Deep in my heart, I knew that running away from intense suffering wouldn't ultimately alleviate it, so I decided to study it instead. I've included an extensive list of my favorite resources on the topic of suffering at the end of this book.

It might seem counterintuitive to spend your time studying something you're trying to get *out* of, but I found this reading and study to be beneficial to my soul. As I read other people's experiences of intense suffering, I learned that this universal experience has spanned the course of history. I found it encouraging to be reminded of the fact that I wasn't the first person to ever experience difficulty, and I wasn't going to be the last. Millions of people have walked through seasons of suffering. Even if their sorrow didn't look exactly like mine, it comforted me to know that nothing surprises God, that He understands the hurting of people throughout the millennia, and that He is present with us through all of it.

Listen to Sacred Music

Many of you may be feeling isolated and alone as you walk through this trial, with seemingly no earthly comfort. But I believe it's there—in one of the darkest pits we'll ever find ourselves—that we truly begin to discover God in a deeper way. While I don't know how long you'll be in the valley, I pray you won't let go of Him. I encourage you to remain firm in your trust of God, refusing to run away from Him, even in your grief. May we hold on to the truth in the old hymn "How Firm a Foundation, Ye Saints of the Lord."

When through the deep waters I call you to go,
The rivers of sorrow shall not overflow,
For I will be with you in trouble to bless,
And sanctify to you your deepest distress.[2]

There's another line from this hymn that I adore:
"That soul, though all hell should endeavor to shake, I'll
never, no, never, no never forsake." Beloved, if you are
God's child, all of hell is laboring against you and tempting you to shift your eyes away from the Lord. The ultimate temptation is to walk away, throw up your hands,
and say, "This is too much. I can't do it. I don't want to do
it." Don't let evil win. Keep wrestling, keep fighting, keep
grieving, but do it all with the Lord. Walking through
this sacred sorrow is the fight of a lifetime. The battle for
belief, the fight for faith, and the war for true womanhood
will be paramount to your relationship with the Lord.

William Cowper was a prolific poet and hymn writer
as well as a friend of John Newton. At the end of his life,
he wrote his most famous song, "God Moves in a Mysterious Way." Cowper's life had been filled with struggles
and difficulties. He suffered through enormous health
challenges and frequent bouts of depression, and he attempted to commit suicide on at least one occasion. What
I appreciate about the life and works of Cowper is the
rich honesty presented in them. He penned hymns with
titles such as "My Soul Is Sad and Much Dismayed" and
"When Darkness Long Has Veiled My Mind."

"God Moves in a Mysterious Way" is supposedly
the last hymn Cowper ever wrote. One evening, the pain
got to be too much, and he decided to commit suicide
by drowning himself. Cowper called a cab and told the

driver to take him to the Thames. As the cabbie drove, a thick fog descended, and he was unable to find the river. After a lot of driving around, the driver stopped and let Cowper out. To his great surprise, he found himself back at his own doorstop.[3]

In the "darkest valley" (NIV), says the psalmist in Psalm 23—and even in a cab with a desperate soul—God, the ever-loving parent, watches over us.

Surround Yourself with a Strong Community

As I've walked through my toughest days, one of the most valuable things has been having tenderhearted friends and family walk with me. If I had to suffer completely alone, I don't think I would have made it through.

I urge you to begin surrounding yourself with people who will lovingly walk through this trial with you. My mom was especially important to me. I have placed hundreds of phone calls for help to her over the years. Time after time, my mom has encouraged me when my faith was too weak, when I felt helpless. She's been there for me in my darkest hours, and she never made me feel like I was asking too much by coming to her constantly for emotional support. Sometimes what we need most is a hug, a listening ear, and a shoulder to cry on.

What kind of person should you invite into this deep suffering with you? Look for someone who will interact with you from a place of tenderness and compassion. Find people who will intentionally ask you how your heart is and aren't afraid of honest and truthful answers. Tears often scare people because they don't know how to react. Find someone who will love you in the midst of tears and pain, someone who is comfortable with difficult and unanswered questions.

Reach out to your church community, ask your pastor to connect you with other men and women. I've found the most helpful companions are those who have experienced deep sorrow themselves. Feel the freedom to avoid those who try to "fix" you or your problems. Perhaps one of God's sweetest blessings to us on this side of eternity is community. We need each other—especially in trying seasons.

Michael Card has written one of the most touching books on suffering I've read. Since he's a songwriter, he has an uncanny way of putting together words and concepts. In his book *A Sacred Sorrow,* he writes so eloquently about lament:

> Our failure to lament also cuts us off from each other. If you and I are to know one another in a deep way, we must not only share our hurts, anger, and disappointments with each other (which we often do), we must also lament them together before the God who hears and is moved by our tears. Only then does our sharing become truly redemptive in character. The degree to which I am willing to enter into the suffering of another person reveals the level of my commitment and love for them. If I am not interested in your hurts, I am not really interested in you. Neither am I willing to suffer to know you nor to be known by you. Jesus' example makes these truths come alive in our hearts. He is the One who suffered to know us, who then suffered for us on the cross.[4]

Read Encouraging Bible Stories

Maybe not all of us need to be taught how to lament, but we need to be given the permission and the freedom to lament. The Bible is filled with the language of lament. Our spiritual forefathers were well acquainted with grief, death, pain, and sorrow. They knew what it meant to cry out, to wrestle, and to bring their raw and unfiltered pain to the Lord. David, Hagar, Jeremiah, Job, Elizabeth, and Jesus are a few of the classic examples of this. Each journeyed on a road paved with sorrow.

It's interesting to note that none of them knew they would be held up throughout the ages as examples in how to suffer well. They never imagined their stories would be recorded in the Holy Scriptures, and except for Jesus, they certainly weren't placed there because of their perfection. In the words of pastor and author Tim Keller in a tweet, "Job never saw why he suffered, but he saw God and that was enough."

Read the Psalms

For the longest time, I tried to tell myself that it would all be okay. That because I believed in God's sovereignty, I should simply accept my sorrows as a part of His sanctifying process. As a result, I didn't allow myself to mourn or truly feel the full weight of the pain. Over the years, I've learned how to lament and grieve before the Lord and with the Lord. I've learned that it's entirely possible to trust in a sovereign God and still be upset, cry, and feel sad.

The nineteenth-century British preacher Charles Spurgeon said, "The sovereignty of God is the pillow upon which the child of God rests his head at night, giving perfect peace."[5] Undergirding all of life, including the excruciatingly difficult things, is the truth that nothing takes God by surprise, and He's in control. As Jerry Bridges says in his excellent book *Trusting God*, "God is infinite in wisdom. God is perfect in love."[6]

That love is illustrated throughout the Bible. Perhaps one of the most important words in the Old Testament is the Hebrew word *hesed*, which does not have a direct correlation in English but is often translated as "loving-kindness, loyalty, mercy, or steadfast love" and describes God's love for us. The word may have a connection—albeit a "doubtful" one—with the Arabic word *hashada*, which means "come together for aid," but the English Bible translation I most appreciate is the word "loyalty."[7]

Nowhere is God's loyal love on greater display than in Psalms where you can see the frequency of this idea expressed:

Psalm 6:4—Turn, O LORD, deliver my life; save me for the sake of your steadfast love.

Psalm 13:5—But I have trusted in your steadfast love; my heart shall rejoice in your salvation.

Psalm 17:7—Wondrously show your steadfast love, O Savior of those who seek refuge from their adversaries at your right hand.

Psalm 25:6—Remember your mercy, O LORD, and your steadfast love, for they have been from of old.

Psalm 26:3—For your steadfast love is before my eyes, and I walk in your faithfulness.

Psalm 31:7—I will rejoice and be glad in your steadfast love, because you have seen my affliction; you have known the distress of my soul.

Psalm 44:26—Rise up; come to our help! Redeem us for the sake of your steadfast love!

Again and again, the psalmists ask God for redemption, aid, protection, and forgiveness. Their entreaties crescendo in Psalm 136 with twenty-six verses that are filled with the refrain "for his steadfast love endures forever." Beloved, you can cling to God's loyal love for you. Along with the chosen people of Israel, you can take comfort in God's promise: "I have loved you with an everlasting love" (Jer. 31:3). His love to us is an unending stream that will sustain us throughout eternity.

"Christian, take this for your comfort," says Charles Spurgeon, "that there is no change in Jesus Christ's love to those who rest in Him. Yesterday you were on Tabor's top, and you said, 'He loves me'; today you are in the valley of humiliation, but He loves you still the same."[8] God views you with a loyal, everlasting love that will never run out no matter how many times you come to Him with your tears, disappointment, and pain.

The Lord will be faithful to you through this desert. It might feel like hope is unattainable right now, but there's no rush to move on to the next step. You're on your own timetable as you process this grief. Don't compare your story to anyone else's. And remember that sorrow and joy can coexist. Katherine Wolf, the author with her husband, Jay, of the excellent book *Hope Heals*, once posted the following on social media: "Good and hard can occupy the exact same space . . . gratitude can be both heavy and light."

The Bible tells us time after time that if we are God's children, suffering is a natural part of our lives. But above everything else, fix your heart on the unchanging fact that the Lord promises never to leave us or forsake us. We can hold on to the truth of Scripture: "The LORD your God is in your midst, a mighty one who will save; he will rejoice over you with gladness; he will quiet you by his love; he will exult over you with loud singing" (Zeph. 3:17).

God's Word has been a huge source of comfort for my frail heart. Other verses I held on to were Joshua 1:5 and 9, Matthew 28:20, and Psalm 23:4. I encourage you to look these verses up, meditate upon them, memorize them, pray them, and cry them out. Squeeze everything you can out of them. You're not alone on this journey through childlessness. I, and many other women, know the heartache you're experiencing. And above anything else, you can rely on God's loyal love, knowing He will be with you every moment.

REFLECTION & DISCUSSION

What are some honest questions you've asked the Lord in your sorrow?

What are some triggers that cause you to get upset?

How can you continue to involve your community in your childlessness?

What music has encouraged your soul?

Choose a few psalms to read every morning. Read them aloud. Write them out. Pray them. Meditate upon them.

How do you see God's grace and love in this chapter?

THREE

TRUSTING GOD'S NO

God's Care in
the Midst of Suffering

*E*ven though learning I could not bear children was my first serious experience with suffering, I've since walked through other trials. Three years ago, my youngest sister fell ill and almost died from a brain condition. Since then, she's endured multiple doctor visits, medications, and attempts to heal her body. Another one of my sisters has had three miscarriages. One of my six siblings isn't a Christian. I've had a major surgery that left me laid up in bed for two weeks, taking as much painkiller as they'd give me.

When these additional disappointments and heartaches came my way, I was admittedly shocked. I found myself wondering, "Haven't I already been through enough heartbreak? Hasn't the Lord given me enough sorrow?" Life often feels like it involves too much hardship, too much pain, and quite honestly, it can feel cruel. I've grieved with friends and sought the Lord, but ultimately I have had to wrestle through another big question: "What do I do when God doesn't change my circumstances?"

It can be so heartbreaking to pray and beg God for something and ask Him to change a situation only to feel like your prayers go unanswered. Even worse is when the Lord says no to some of your deepest desires. What do you do when this happens? How do you reconcile unanswered prayers with the truth of God's sovereignty and goodness? If we're honest with ourselves, we're worried that He won't come through for us. We've been disappointed one too many times, and we're scared to trust Him. Despite our longings to have a baby, our circumstances seem to demonstrate that God can't be trusted because we don't have what we have begged and pleaded for. We begin questioning God, asking, "God, if You're all-powerful, why aren't You fixing this?" Certainly, He's able to give us our desires and remove the trials from our lives, but He sometimes chooses not to.

I was raised in a Christian household and my parents are two of the strongest, godliest people I've ever known. As a young child, I prayed to accept Christ as my Savior and tried to get to know Him and follow Him. Growing up, I was the good girl, always seeking to please my parents and other authority figures in my life. I was rewarded for my good behavior, and I learned that if I worked hard enough and was "good" enough I could get what I wanted, be successful, and achieve my goals. Life was pretty straightforward: my hard work + my goodness = success.

During my teenage years, my family went through some financial difficulties that almost threatened to undo us. Some days were pretty scary, including the time the power was shut off at home and we didn't have the money to turn it back on immediately. We ended up going to my dad's office that evening and eating peanut butter sandwiches while my parents figured out what the next step was. This season was my first encounter with hardship, but none of it was my fault, and there was nothing I could do to make it better. So, while it affected me emotionally, I still felt safe because I was in my parents' care and deep down knew we'd be okay. As a family, we grew closer together, pinched every penny, and made it through those lean years.

But I didn't experience a personal crisis of faith until I found out I was barren. I've never been closer to walking away from God. If I'm being completely honest, I went through a season where I had to sit down and think through whether I wanted to follow Christ. My cross felt too heavy to bear. I was weary, angry, and grieving.

Today, I can look back at that family financial crisis and see it as a beautiful metaphor for God's loving, parental care. During that time, I didn't worry while sitting in the darkness, I was grateful for our simple meal, and I didn't compare my circumstances to anyone else's. All I knew was to look to my father, because I knew he loved me, and I trusted who he was.

Despite our circumstances, let's look to the truth.

THE LIFELINE OF THE SOUL

Have you ever been tempted in moments of extreme difficulty to throw up your hands and say, "It's not worth it.

God isn't worth it"? It was in those raw moments that I found myself praying the most honest prayers of my life. I was in the fire, and prayer wasn't just a nice sentiment, it became the lifeline of my soul. Nestled atop a hill on Liberty's campus was a small white chapel. The picturesque building became home to some deep lament. I'm an introvert and often needed to escape the noise and chatter that constantly surrounded me. The little chapel was the quietest place I could find, and I escaped to its musty, dimly lit sanctuary. It always took a moment to adjust my eyes as I entered. There were never more than a handful of people praying there at one time, and I gravitated toward my favorite pew—middle, right side—my Bible in hand. I usually started off my time by reading a few psalms. The honesty of the prayers in that book provided the language I needed to express my heart to God. I learned how to pray in that chapel and how to persevere, even in the most trying times.

Our souls often need space and quietness to begin actually feeling and processing. Throughout the psalms, we learn that many of the authors often cried and grieved during the nighttime: "I am weary with my moaning; every night I flood my bed with tears; I drench my couch with my weeping. My eye wastes away because of grief" (Ps. 6:6–7). And again in Psalm 22:1–2: "My God, my God, why have you forsaken me? Why are you so far from saving me, from the words of my groaning? O my God, I cry by day, but you do not answer, and by night, but I find no rest."

Some of Jesus' most intimate times of prayer were at night, and He even chose to spend His last night on earth in prayer. The wee hours of the night are often the only time we truly have the quiet we need to begin feeling and expressing those feelings to the Lord. It can be easy to stuff our feelings down to merely survive our busy days. Beginning to pray those honest prayers, to contend with the Lord in prayer, to tell Him how you're feeling and holding nothing back, those are vital steps in walking with the Lord when you don't understand your circumstances or God's plan.

GOD'S CONSTANT CARE

For the first time in my life, my good behavior wasn't gaining me a blessing. It is so easy to slip into thinking that if you're a Christian, you are immune from trials. Surely if God loved us, He would bless us. Right? We find ourselves making statements like the following:

> If God really loved me, He wouldn't have allowed _____ into my life.

> If God really loved me, He wouldn't have taken _____ from me.

> If God really loved me, He wouldn't withhold a good thing from me.

> If God really loved me, He would give me children.

This kind of flawed thinking started all the way back in Genesis, when the crafty serpent whispered into Eve's ear, "Did God actually say. . . ?" (Gen. 3:1). Skillfully, he caused her to doubt everything she knew to be true and to question every promise the Lord had made to her and Adam. We aren't told if this scene took place over the course of a few hours or a few weeks. Did Eve wrestle and weigh the consequences of her actions? Or did she make a quick judgment call, longing so strongly for the good she thought God was withholding from her that she was willing to say yes to momentary pleasure? We don't know; but we do know the rest of the story all too well:

> When the woman saw that the fruit of the tree was good for food and pleasing to the eye, and also desirable for gaining wisdom, she took some and ate it. She also gave some to her husband, who was with her, and he ate it. Then the eyes of both of them were opened, and they realized they were naked; so they sewed fig leaves together and made coverings for themselves. (Gen. 3:6–7 NIV)

Interestingly enough, a part of the curse that the Lord placed upon the woman was to multiply her pain in childbearing. Sin changed everything, including women's bodies. Perhaps Eve believed that if God really loved her, He wouldn't withhold this good food from her; regardless, her decision had devastating consequences.

Recently, my former college roommate, who is also one of my best friends, moved back into the area where I live. Eagerly, we scheduled dinner to catch up on life. So much had happened during the few years we'd been apart, including Lauren having three miscarriages before finally giving birth to her daughter. When we met up, it felt as if no time had passed, and we were able to quickly slip back into deep and intimate conversation. Lauren and I chatted about the sweet things we'd seen the Lord do in our lives but also poured out our hearts about the difficult paths we'd walked.

The conversation inevitably turned to the three little babies she and her husband had lost. With tears in her eyes, Lauren began to tell me about miscarriage after miscarriage. By the time she reached the third one, it felt like my heart was going to break. Lauren told me that she knew the Lord was all powerful and able to breathe life into her babies, saving their lives. But after the third loss, she was at her wits' end and began questioning why God didn't change her circumstances. She explained to me that her initial reaction was to grapple with the Lord with a frustrated and angry heart.

Many of us, when encountering a difficult circumstance for the first time, begin an epic wrestling match with the Lord. Often we've been denied our heart's desire, so we begin to bargain with Him.

"God, if You allow me to have children, I promise I'll dedicate them to You."

"God, if You make me a mother, I'll love and serve You all my days."

"God, don't You realize that unbelievers will be able to see Your goodness if You answer this prayer?"

I shared at the beginning of this book that when I began to tell friends that I couldn't have my own children, several people questioned my level of faith and wondered if I had prayed enough. "Surely you must have done something wrong. Examine your own heart." The hurtful words that were spoken reminded me of the story of the blind man in John 9. The disciples were walking with Jesus when they passed by a man who'd been blind since birth. Inquisitively, the disciples asked Jesus, "Rabbi, who sinned, this man or his parents, that he was born blind?" Jesus answered, "It was not that this man sinned, or his parents, but that the works of God might be displayed in him" (John 9:2–3). Even the disciples easily fell into believing that God's favor followed God's favorites.

Though these friends and acquaintances meant well, their comments were detrimental to my walk with the Lord. More than likely, someone has uttered similar sentiments to you. Quietly, in the stillness of your heart, you begin to think there's something wrong with you. These doubts and questions echo the lies the devil whispered to Eve in paradise. Satan caused Eve to attempt to solve her own problems and perceived lack, rather than resting in the truth that God had already given her and Adam everything they needed. They were in paradise, walking and talking with God Almighty! What more could they need? But the devil tricked Eve into thinking that God was withholding good from her.

GOD'S WAYS ARE DIFFERENT THAN OURS

We must also be on our guard against so-called biblical teaching that promises that God will give us whatever we desire, long, and hope for. The sentiment that God will reward our good behavior with blessing upon blessing is found nowhere in the Bible and perpetuates a wholly inadequate and unbiblical view of the relationship between God and human beings. What you believe about God dictates how you interact with God. The simple fact is that we are not guaranteed perfection here on earth, despite what many prominent speakers and authors promise. The biblical gospel is God-centered, not human-centered.

As it says in Matthew, "If anyone would come after

me, let him deny himself and take up his cross and follow me" (Matt. 16:24). We shouldn't be following Christ for the earthly blessings we can gain. "For what does it profit a man to gain the whole world and forfeit his soul?" (Mark 8:36). In fact, I've found that trials have a way of revealing where our hearts are, where we've been placing our trust, and where we've been seeking joy, hope, and security. These are the questions we should be asking ourselves:

> "Will I continue to trust God even if He never fulfills my earthly desire?"
>
> "Will I continue to follow God even if He never reveals the purpose for my suffering?"
>
> "Will I cling to the fact that God loves me even if I don't always feel it?"

God *is* sovereign and all-powerful. Although He has the power to instantly change a circumstance, He's working for different purposes that are often beyond our understanding. He's weaving all the strands of history together to make a masterpiece so magnificent that only eternity will fully reveal His plans. The respected theologian D. A. Carson writes, "It does help to know that there is light at the end of the tunnel, even if you cannot yet see it; to know that God is in control and is committed to his people's good, even though it still does not look like that to you. The suffering is no less real, but perhaps it is less debilitating when the larger perspective is kept in mind."[1]

The Bible is chock-full of people who walked through dark experiences, shattered dreams, and unfulfilled desires.

If you focus only on the stark circumstances of their lives, it might seem as if God was absent or that He didn't care enough to answer their prayers. Just take a look at this short list:

Adam and Eve were thrown out of paradise. (Gen. 3:23–24)

Abraham and Sarah struggled with infertility for twenty-five years. (Gen. 11:30; 21:1–6)

Rachel was infertile for a number of years. (Gen. 29:31)

Leah was consistently overlooked since Jacob loved Rachel more. (Gen. 29:30)

Joseph was unfairly imprisoned. (Gen 39:20)

Job lost loved ones, possessions, and almost everything he held dear. (Book of Job)

Mary watched her oldest son be crucified. (John 19:16–27)

Paul endured tremendous personal trials including a shipwreck, beatings, and imprisonment. (Acts 21:27–36; 2 Cor. 11:23–30)

JESUS, THE GREAT EMPATHIZER

We have the privilege of reading the Bible cover to cover, so we know the end of the stories listed above. We can see that the Lord was quietly working in the background, orchestrating a grand narrative that reveals His glory. There is no question that experiencing unfulfilled longings or unmet desires is difficult. And sometimes our communities do not do a very good job of creating space for us to grieve the things that have been lost.

In spite of that, we must remember that Jesus was called the Man of Sorrows. He knew what it meant to cry, and not one of our tears falls without His noticing or caring (see Ps. 56:8). Jesus saw the world as it is, broken and sinful and grieving. We tend to skim over the fact that Jesus had feelings, that He experienced sadness, anger, and frustration. Perhaps we sometimes fail to remember that Jesus was fully human. He suffered in a way we can't comprehend and in a way that no one else ever has or will: death on a cross while bearing the sins of the world. When you feel as if God doesn't love you, look to the cross. God loves you. We might not get everything we want in this life—few of us do—but I can assure you that the Father cares deeply for you.

My mom has told me hundreds of times that she wishes she could take my pain on herself. If she could, she'd take all my hardships in an instant. When she first began to tell me this, I thought, "That's nice of you to say, but you *can't* take my pain away." Only perfect love could speak those words. As time passed, I learned to understand that she was communicating, "Chelsea, I love you so much that I want to bear your burdens instead of you." Her love was pointing me toward a greater love— God's love. While no human can ever take away our pain, they can help ease it.

Trying to trick you into thinking that God doesn't love you is one of Satan's oldest and dirtiest tricks. Satan wants to hurt God as much as possible, and what better way to hurt Him than to hurt His children? If God didn't love you, He wouldn't have sent His only Son to take on His wrath. If God didn't love you, He wouldn't have made promises in His Word. The famous German pastor Dietrich Bonhoeffer reminds us that "God does not give us everything we want, but He does fulfill His promises, leading us along the best and straightest paths to Himself."[2]

Since childlessness was the first trial that hit me hard, I was not only grieving the loss of my dream to carry my own babies, I was also learning how to truly grieve. For the first time in my life, I didn't get what I most wanted, and I didn't know how to handle it. In a book written on another one of life's heartaches—the act of suicide—Albert Hsu explains both the universality of grief, for both the believer and nonbeliever:

> Christians sometimes think that we are not supposed to grieve, because our faith and theology provide us with confidence about heaven and eternal life. But while 1 Thessalonians 4:13 says that we are not to grieve as those without hope, we grieve nevertheless. Those without hope grieve in one way; those with hope grieve in another. Either way, grief is universal and not to be avoided. It is a legitimate response to loss.[3]

Our emotions and feelings aren't something we should try to hide or ignore. The Lord created emotions to be expressed. Emotions of sadness and anger are an indicator that something is not right. Nancy Guthrie, an author and Bible teacher, has ministered to my soul through her writing. She communicates with a tenderness toward the suffering and writes out of her experiences of losing two children as infants. With a deep understanding of this trial, she reminds us that "tears do not reflect a lack of faith . . . tears are a gift from God that help to wash away the deep pain of loss."[4] Don't be afraid of your tears. Feel those emotions deeply. Truly grieving and stepping into the sacred sorrow is a prerequisite for walking through the rest of this journey, especially while carrying the realization that the Lord sometimes doesn't change our circumstances.

As I began to come to terms with the fact that I'd never have my own children, I was faced with a choice. How was I going to respond when God didn't give me what I wanted? What was I going to do? What was I going to say? All my life I'd heard that God was enough, but now I was going to have to choose whether or not I actually believed that. For me, this decision process was a slow one.

As you live through this season of sorrow and wrestle through your pain and questions, you'll begin to see that God *is* enough. You will come to proclaim with St. Augustine: "You have made us for Yourself, O Lord, and our heart is restless until it finds its rest in You." We were created specifically and intentionally for God and nothing on earth can truly satisfy our hearts like His presence.

We learn in the book of Job about a godly man whose life was wrecked by trials. Job lost his wealth, his children, and his health, all while interacting with friends who questioned his righteousness and looked for something to blame for his suffering. Like Job, we have a choice to make: What will our reaction be when the Lord withholds apparent good from us or when we suffer traumatic events? I used to think my reaction had to be immediate worship.

All my life I'd been taught good theology, and I knew the right responses to almost any question. But what I didn't yet have was a theology of suffering, since I didn't have any personal experience with it. We might know with our minds that the Lord is good, sovereign, powerful, loving, kind, and strong. But when we walk through difficult life experiences that argue the exact opposite, what are we going to do?

CHILDREN AREN'T OUR RIGHT

Jean E. Jones, author of *Discovering Hope in the Psalms* (a book that has deeply ministered to me), started following Christ early in her life. In high school, she started teaching a Bible study and leading other women into a closer relationship with their Father. After she met and married her husband, Clay, they never expected the heartbreak that was in store for them. Miscarriage after miscarriage caused them to examine what they believed about their faith. After the fifth miscarriage, Jean recalls her crying out to the Lord in her pain and the answer God gave her.

> Everyone else can have children—why can't I? . . . As soon as those words came out of my mouth, I knew I'd misspoken. Many women cannot have children; some also have no husband. Then it hit me: I'd felt entitled to motherhood. This was the root of my anger. I felt God had denied me a "right." . . . At that moment, I realized all of life involves choosing between conflicting desires. Our choices reveal what we value most. I suddenly understood sacrificial praise (Heb. 13:15) in

a new way: choosing to praise and glorify God by relinquishing something costly. I wanted to offer sacrificial praise, but finding the words was hard.[5]

Jones presents an interesting perspective: bearing children isn't a guaranteed right, it's a gift. Even though I believe the longing to have children is a godly desire, the Lord doesn't always give us the things we most desire. Elisabeth Elliot once prayed, "Oh Lord, give me that which I desire, or teach my heart how to long for something better." Following Jesus is costly.

Vaneetha Rendall Risner, another dear sister in the faith and author of *The Scars That Have Shaped Me*, lost a child at a young age because of a doctor's mistake. She's written prolifically on the subject of suffering and has some powerful words to say about the influence of the story of Job on her outlook:

> Ironically, it was the book of Job that had helped me reframe my perspective on God's blessings. *I saw that naming what we want and then claiming the victory is not worshipping God. It is idolatry. The focus is not on God but rather on what He can give us.* It's elevating God's gifts above Him, the giver. And that is a great assault on God's value.[6]

Even though I've never met any of these women personally, their words have profoundly influenced me. Instead of focusing so much on what I lack, these reminders helped me lift my head up and begin to see God in the midst of the pain. By meditating on these truths, I was able to slowly begin shifting my perspective. A few months into my childlessness, I began to pray that the Lord would teach me how to long for Him more than I longed for a child. When I first started to pray that prayer, I felt like I was getting nowhere. Months went by and the pain just seemed to intensify. I was so confused and prayed, "God, I don't understand! I want to want You more than I want a baby. But You aren't taking away that longing. Why?" In my pain, I continued to seek Him.

It wasn't a pretty sight; it was raw and real. I was expecting God to change my heart dramatically and remove my desire for motherhood. I thought, "If God is going to teach me how to focus on Him instead of a blessing, surely, He'll take away my longings so I'll have even more room in my heart for Him." What I wasn't understanding was that my longings were the very things He was using to teach me reliance on Him. I begged Him to remove my weakness, but He used it to draw me closer to Himself.

Even though years have passed since my diagnosis, I *still* have a longing in my heart for a child. Over time, I've learned that having longings isn't bad. How I choose to respond to the longings is what matters, and I have two choices in those moments. First, I can dwell on the longing and what I lack. My heart can become obsessed with the good I think God is withholding from me, and I can become angry and bitter. Or I can take those longings to God and allow Him to comfort me and teach me.

How we respond to suffering says something to the world about God. If we had everything we wanted, there would never be a reason to trust God and the world would not see that our God truly is big enough, kind enough, and good enough to walk with us even on the roads we would never select for ourselves. We can properly grieve, but as Christians we grieve with our ultimate hope resting in Christ. Jesus secured our redemption on the cross, but it didn't come without a price. The call to follow our victorious Savior is ultimately a call to die to our desires and our flesh in order to truly, deeply live. The paradox of Christian suffering is that we are refined in the fires of adversity. While I would never have chosen this enormous pain for my life, my heart is closer to God because of it. I pray that whatever darkness you're walking through, you will cling to the truth that God's grace is sufficient for you (see 2 Cor. 12:9).

It's such a human response to think, "If God really did love me, He'd give me what I want." If we're honest with ourselves and the Lord, we blame God when He seems to withhold good gifts from us or appears to take away good things. There will be times when the Lord does not answer our prayers in the way we expect, and sometimes He tells His children no. Sometimes He reveals the reasons why, but many times we will not understand this side of heaven. I still grieve because God hasn't redeemed my trials or fulfilled all my longings. If I allow myself to linger in that place for too long, I'll slip into despair. We must remember that we can't always look to our circumstances as evidence of God's love for us. It's so natural and easy to tie God's goodness to what He chooses to give us, but that's a false gospel.

Second Peter 1:3 tell us, "His divine power has granted to us all things that pertain to life and godliness." If we lack something, perhaps God does not consider it a true necessity. God's definition of need and ours is often different. Or as Tim Keller reminds us, "If Jesus is God, then he's got to be great enough to have some reasons to let you go through things you can't understand."[7]

YOUR TRIAL HAS AN END DATE

Though it might not feel like it right now, this struggle is temporary. More than any other person, Charles Spurgeon has helped me fix my eyes on God. His writing and preaching possess a tenderness that only could have been learned by going through the fire. Throughout his life, Spurgeon struggled with depression and dark nights of the soul. Even though written in the midst of his suffering, his words remind us still today of a powerful truth.

> Our sorrows are all, like ourselves, mortal. There are no immortal sorrows for immortal souls. They come, but blessed be God, they also go. Like birds of the air, they fly over our heads. But they cannot make their abode in our souls. We suffer today, but we shall rejoice tomorrow.[8]

I still remember the exact moment when I learned that my trial has an end date. Growing up, I was close to my Greek next-door neighbors and was invited to spend a few weeks with them in Greece. I immediately accepted and found myself in Athens in the middle of summer. A few days into my trip, I was taking a rest period during the hottest part of the afternoon. I slipped out to the balcony surrounded by beauty and started to cry. I was overcome with homesickness, and all I wanted to do was hop on a plane and head back to North Carolina to be with my mom and dad. Instead, I flipped open my Bible hoping to find comfort there. I landed in Revelation 21, as I read the first few verses, I felt hope well up in my heart.

> Then I saw new heaven and a new earth, for the first heaven and the first earth had passed away, and the sea was no more. And I saw the holy city, new Jerusalem, coming down out of heaven from God, prepared as a bride adorned for her husband. And I heard a loud voice from the throne saying, "Behold, the dwelling place of God is with man. He will dwell with them, and they will be his people, and God himself will be with them as their God. He will wipe away every tear from their eyes, and death shall be no more, neither shall there be mourning, nor crying, nor pain anymore, for the former things have passed away." (Rev. 21:1–4)

Verse 2 is one of the most stunning verses in the Bible: "Behold, the dwelling place of God is with man." The King who created the world, the Savior who died for us despite our sin, the Holy Spirit who dwells in us—this Trinitarian God chooses to dwell with His people. And the culmination of this epic love story will be in eternity when we finally are united with Him. God promises to be with us forever. We can stake our hope in that claim.

I know it may not feel like it, but one day this trial will end. One day the Lord will wipe away all your sorrow and your sadness. Cling to that promise with everything in you. While we aren't guaranteed our best life now, we have a future hope we can cling to.

The *hesed* of God is yours forever. It's possible to

thrive and be fully alive while still hurting. The two can coexist. Of course I'm not trying to say that if you fix your eyes on heaven, all your earthly sorrows will disappear. Obviously, they won't. But one day, all the horrible pain and suffering you've experienced will be a distant memory. Hold on and trust that though your heavenly Father might not change your circumstances, He's transforming you to look more like Him. That's more precious than anything He could ever give us.

REFLECTION & DISCUSSION

How do you respond when you don't get what you want?

Have you been tempted to believe that God's care for you is directly tied to His blessing to you? If so, what are some ways you can begin to change your perspective?

In what ways can you cultivate quietness in your heart, to allow yourself space to pray and talk honestly with the Lord?

How have you seen and experienced God's fatherly care for you, even in the midst of suffering?

How can you remind yourself that your trials have an expiration date?

How do you see God's grace and love in this chapter?

FOUR

GRIEVING YOUR UNFULFILLED DESIRE
Childless Women
Who Found Hope

*U*nfulfilled longings and desires, unmet expectations, and shattered dreams are hard to face. It feels like getting a bucket of cold water dumped on your head. As I've been writing this book, Michael and I have been watching *Planet Earth II*. I'm absolutely fascinated with nature—one of my favorite places to be and one of my favorite things to study. It's so easy to see God's handiwork. I'm amazed by the stunning care and creativity with which the Lord designed the earth. But I'm also struck by the fact that each animal reproduces while I, a human woman, am incapable of bearing a child. Even the animals are more successful than I am in this area.

As we continue taking steps toward finding real and solid hope, we need to camp out here a bit longer in grief. If we rush too quickly through the grieving process, we won't be able to move forward with the rest of our lives. We never "get over" the death of a child or an inability to bear children. Those types of heartaches stay with us. Rightly so, because this trial is excruciatingly difficult. However, I believe it is possible to process the pain in a healthy way so we can embrace our future.

What is grief? Grief is a natural response to loss, and I believe grief is a God-given emotional response when things aren't the way they should be. As time passed, I learned that it was okay not to be okay. For so long, I tried to grit my teeth and make it through pain. This ended up backfiring. Because I wasn't carefully tending to my needs and emotions, I ended up a wreck. You don't have to always be brave or strong. Press into the pain, and allow yourself to fully feel it. It will hurt tremendously, but grieving is good for the soul.

When I first found out that I was barren, I'd find myself grieving at the most unpredictable times. As the weeks passed, I learned what things triggered my grief and how to begin controlling those triggers. For example, I'd try to avoid being around children for too long, because it served as a reminder of what I didn't have. Months flew by, and I still found my grief frequently rising to the surface; however, I began to push it back down and move on with my day. Feeling all these feelings was inconvenient and hindered my ability to live life. Desperate to stop living like this and feeling like I'd hit rock bottom, I did the only thing I could think of. I reached out to a counselor. Taking care of my mental health was not something

I'd been taught. I just knew I hated how often I was still getting upset and crying and how difficult life was to live. I needed help.

I'd had a stigma about counseling in my mind, largely because I didn't grow up knowing anyone who went to counseling. I assumed it was for weak people who couldn't handle life on their own. But I reached a point where I needed help, and I sheepishly reached out to the counselor at Liberty. My first visit in her office was awkward, embarrassing, and stressful. I found myself sitting on a sofa in a softly lit room with a stranger asking me too many personal questions. As the weeks passed, she helped me begin processing through my unfulfilled desires. Most of our sessions were spent with her asking me lots of questions and my talking through my emotions. Since she was a Christian, she directed me to the Bible. We spent a lot of time chatting through the childless women in Scripture, and what lessons I would come to learn from them!

Notably, there are several prominent stories in the Bible that feature women who struggled with childlessness. How did these women respond when their bodies wouldn't bear babies? For me, the most vivid story of barrenness is Hannah's story, found in 1 Samuel. In that time, it was customary for men to take multiple wives. Elkanah was married to both Hannah and Peninnah. Seemingly, the most important part of their story is children, or lack thereof. Peninnah had children, while Hannah remained barren. *The MacArthur Study Bible* suggests that Elkanah married Peninnah because Hannah was barren. Peninnah was likely the second wife, but the first to bear children.[1] I can only imagine how difficult this was for Hannah! Throughout the opening verses of this chapter, we learn of Hannah's struggle, and we're told that she wept bitterly, refused to eat, was deeply distressed, filled with anxiety, and vexed (see 1 Samuel 1:3–11). In addition to her barrenness, Peninnah—whom the Bible refers to as Hannah's rival—would provoke and irritate her, constantly reminding her of what she lacked—fertility. Hannah's own heartbreak was surely compounded by the expectations of women in the ancient world, which equated bearing children with God's blessing.[2] Is it any wonder, then, that these displays of tears and emotions were Hannah's response? She was grieving.

I'm so encouraged that the Lord chose to include this story in the Bible, because it reminds us that childlessness is indeed a trial and is worth mourning. Through these stories, we see that God is present in this trial and that He cares about those experiencing it. These biblical examples also teach us that our natural emotional reaction should not be downplayed or quashed. We were created with tears and with emotions for a reason.

We see that Hannah responded by pouring out her soul to the Lord, making a solemn vow that if God would give her a son, she would dedicate him to the Lord (1 Sam. 1:11). And the Lord was indeed gracious to Hannah, whose very name means grace. "The LORD remembered her. And in due time Hannah conceived and bore a son" (1 Sam. 1:19–20). Even if He'd chosen to act in a different way, our heavenly Father is worthy of our faith and trust. And because the rest of the story is told in the Bible, we get to see how God's plan for that child unfolded and that Samuel became a prophet of the Lord.

The Bible is filled with imperfect people—people who doubted frequently, whose lives were littered with mistakes, and above all else, people who were honest in their reactions and emotional responses. No one in the Bible ever trusted the Lord fully except Jesus; everyone else stumbled and failed, just like you and me.

Another story of childlessness in the Bible is the story of Abraham and Sarah. Soon after learning the genealogy of Shem in Genesis 11, we are introduced to Abram and his wife, Sarai, who "was barren; she had no child" (Gen. 11:30). Sarai's first reaction was to try to take matters into her own hands. As the years wore on, she doubted that she'd get pregnant, so she tried to manipulate circumstances in order for Abram to have a child. God intervened in their story, and we witness Abram's dramatic calling and the Lord's promise to him and his descendants: "I will make of you a great nation, and I will bless you and make your name great, so that you will be a blessing" (Gen. 12:2).

Have you wondered what Abram and Sarai might have been thinking? Sarai was barren, yet the Lord was promising to make them a great nation. What a stretch it must have been to take God at His word! In fact, they would endure many more years of barrenness before they finally received the son they so desperately longed for. But God, despite their doubts and unbelief, delivered on His promise in spectacular fashion. Finally, in Genesis chapter 21, even though old age was starting to catch up with them both, "the LORD visited Sarah as he had said, and the LORD did to Sarah as he had promised. And Sarah conceived and bore Abraham a son in his old age at the time of which God had spoken to him" (21:1–2). Abraham and Sarah lived through the heartache of childlessness, yet they experience profound redemption and the fulfillment of God's promises to them. Likewise, I and other women like Sarah, have discovered that our emotions, especially our grief, are not too big for God.

Karly is one such woman. To an outsider, it might appear she has everything—beauty, a handsome husband, and—now—a beautiful little boy. Before conceiving and giving birth to this child, Karly had become pregnant with their first child, and she and her husband eagerly began to plan for a big family. But tragedy struck a few months later when Karly had a miscarriage. The couple was completely heartbroken, and Karly cried for days. She said that when the baby's heart stopped beating and the baby was taken from her arms, a piece of her and her husband was gone forever. Despite pleading and bargaining with God, they still lost their child. Karly found great solace in taking all her raw emotions to the Lord and refused to walk away from Him. Her response mirrored the faith of Abraham and Sarah as she kept following the Lord and never lost sight of who He is.

Everyone's journey with childlessness looks different, but regardless of how yours looks, the result (whether temporary or permanent) is the same. You don't have a baby. There's a hole in your heart over what's missing, and it's right and healthy to mourn the loss. Recall how Hannah and Sarah responded; they wept, cried out, and mourned. As we study the lives of Bible characters who experienced childlessness, it's inspiring to see how they trusted the Lord to love them—protests, questions, emotions, and all. They raised their voices and grieved.

There's a key difference between Sarah's and Hannah's grieving and ours today: the church. The childless women we read about in the Old Testament didn't have the church to love, support, and encourage them as they experienced barrenness. We have the incredible blessing of living within the context of a local church. The church, when it recognizes and accepts the call, gets to walk with us in our grief.

Although there are guiding principles in grieving, there is no "one size fits all" path or process.[3] Certified death educator and counselor Dr. Earl Grollman says, "Grief is not a disorder, a disease, or a sign of weakness. It is an emotional, physical, and spiritual necessity, the price you pay for love. The only cure for grief is to grieve."[4]

During my own grieving process, I discovered some of the myths that exist about grieving. It will be helpful, both for those who are grieving and for those who are trying to help, to take a closer look at these myths.

MYTH #1
THE PAIN WILL GO AWAY
FASTER IF YOU IGNORE IT.

Suppressing your pain will only make it worse in the long run. In fact, not allowing yourself to express that pain may cause damage not only to your mind and soul but also to your body.[5] My panic attacks were a prime example of this. In addition, I found myself getting sick frequently, because I wasn't properly taking care of my health or releasing my grief. A major part of the healing process is actually facing your loss head-on and actively dealing with it, instead of pretending it doesn't exist. As the months went on, I tried to suppress the pain that was in my heart. I thought that if I ignored the pain, it wouldn't hurt me as much. My carefully constructed plan backfired, and I found myself worse off than if I'd faced the pain head-on. If I'd allowed myself to grieve when I felt sad instead of stuffing my feelings, I think I could have avoided some major breakdowns and pitfalls along the way.

Be willing to feel your pain, instead of suppressing it. It might hurt more in the short run, but it will help the healing process. Invite the people in your life to help you slow down, process, and mourn.

MYTH #2
IF YOU DON'T CRY, IT MEANS
YOU'RE NOT SAD ABOUT YOUR LOSS.

Grief takes on many forms. Though tears can be one response, crying is not the only one. You may have a different way of showing your grief, in general, or you're just "all cried out." Some people silently mourn their loss, and others turn to friends to talk out their feelings. Just because you might not cry all the time doesn't mean that you don't feel things as deeply as others. I've seen people try to over-compensate in different areas of their life, which usually ends up being harmful. This can play itself out in border-line addictive behaviors such as focusing on perfectionism in an area of your life that you feel like you can control.

Don't put pressure on yourself to grieve a certain way. If you aren't a crier, that's okay. Choose outlets for your grief that are healthful and pleasing to God. I love to put on classical music and spend an afternoon painting. I'm not any good, but I don't care. I do it because it gives me space to express what I'm feeling. For you, that may be having someone sit quietly with you or taking a long walk on a pretty day. Whatever it is, allow yourself the space and time to feed your soul.

Grieve in a way that is comfortable for you.

MYTH #3
GRIEF SHOULD ONLY LAST
FOR A CERTAIN AMOUNT OF TIME.

Despite what you might hear, there is no standard mourning period. Especially if you are grieving a significant loss and depending on your circumstances, grieving can take weeks or even years.[6] Don't box yourself into a time frame or tell yourself that you need to be done grieving by a certain date. "Don't rush the process," says Christina Fox in her article "Helping the Hurting," explaining:

> After a certain amount of time has passed, we might think our friend should have moved on from grief or sorrow . . . But some trials linger with people for much of their lives. We need to stick with them for the long haul. Sometimes our loved one may seem to be doing well, and then something triggers the pain and grief all over again. We need to remember the great patience and forbearance God has for us and provide the same for our friends.[7]

Remember that you have all the time you need to grieve. Give yourself grace to ask for time and to take ample time.

MYTH #4
EVERYONE GRIEVES THE SAME WAY.

Many people are familiar with the five stages of grief, which describes an orderly process of denial, anger, bargaining, depression, and acceptance. However, many grief therapists now tell us that grief is as personal and unique as a fingerprint. Each person is built differently, and we should expect them to grieve differently.

Don't box yourself in with how you respond to unfulfilled desire. Since everyone is different, everyone's response to grief will be different. The way you grieve may not be the same way other women experiencing similar trials grieve.

MYTH #5
MOVING ON WITH YOUR LIFE MEANS
FORGETTING ABOUT YOUR LOSS.

In all likelihood, you'll be reminded in some fashion for the rest of your life of what you lost or what you don't have. In spite of that, it's important to continue taking steps toward renewed life and healing. Just because you're seeking hope doesn't mean you've forgotten your loss.

Once you do come to a place where you feel like you've begun healing, press into that. Your loss will always be a part of your story, but you have the freedom to heal from your pain.

Even though your church, friends, or family may never know the depth of your grief, the Lord sees you. The One who created you understands, and He loves and cares for you. Praise the Lord we have a God who grieved!

I love the way that David and the other psalmists grieved as well. The book of Psalms is filled with their cries, groans, and complaints. From one of the best known, Psalm 23, we learn how to grieve as a Christian while still praising and trusting our Lord: "Even though I walk through the valley of the shadow of death, I will fear no evil, for you are with me; your rod and your staff, they comfort me" (Ps. 23:4). Grief is messy, raw, and real. I find it significant that the Bible includes these pictures of grief and grace. That serves us well as we deal with pain and loss.

So, how then should we grieve? Many of us are taught that prayer, Scripture reading, meditation, and silence are all spiritual disciplines. Even though these practices are critical for spiritual growth, there are times when grieving itself can function as a spiritual discipline. According to evangelist and author Donald Whitney, a characteristic of a spiritual discipline is that it's an activity, not an attitude. It's something you do. He refers to spiritual disciplines that are biblical being "practices taught or modeled in the Bible."[8]

Oh, how well grief fits this definition. Why then are we so quick to overlook it in the church? Maybe it's because grief isn't black and white; because it's not as predictable or tangible as the other spiritual disciplines. We need to be taught that we can lament and grieve. Our hearts need to be shepherded through grief instead of avoiding it. And our churches need to provide the space and freedom for us to do this. One of the best things the church can do to practically provide this kind of support is remembering that grief is a process. It's going to be hard, it's going to be messy, and it's going to be worth it.

In 1 Samuel, Hannah's prayers became so fervent that Eli the priest thought she was drunk. When Eli questioned her about her supposed drunkenness, she was honest and forthright: "No, my lord, I am a woman troubled in spirit. I have drunk neither wine nor strong drink, but I have been pouring out my soul before the LORD" (1 Sam. 1:15). Hannah was grieving. Rachel gave voice to her longing for children by crying out to her husband, Jacob: "Give me children, or I shall die!" (Gen. 30:1). Throughout Scripture, we see the most sorrowful people pouring out their souls before the Lord. Job cried out to the Lord with transparency, "I cry to you for help and you do not answer me; I stand, and you only look at me. You have turned cruel to me; with the might of your hand you persecute me. You lift me up on the wind; you make me ride on it, and you toss me about in the roar of the storm" (Job 30:20–22).

While the emotions we experience during grief are valid, and we can go to God *with* them, part of learning to lament is remembering that our emotions shouldn't *rule* us.

I found that learning to lament and grieve best involves these practices:

Pray with Honesty

When grieving, it is imperative to *pray*. Tim Keller reminds us of this in his book *Prayer*: "Our prayers should arise out of immersion in the Scripture . . . The wedding of the Bible and prayer anchors your life down in the real God."[9] Beloved, it's okay to be honest with the Lord about your circumstances and about your grief. You don't have to hide your true feelings when you approach the throne in prayer. God is waiting for you with open arms, ready to embrace and comfort you.

Cultivate Gratitude

Though it may seem counterintuitive, I encourage you to cultivate gratitude in the midst of your grief. Even though you're walking a dark and dismal road, there are things you can be grateful for. You might have to fight hard to find them. They may be small and seemingly insignificant gifts such as air filling your lungs, an encouraging word from a friend, the beauty of a sunset, or the sight of a bright robin outside your kitchen window. Even though it might not be obvious, everything in your life is a gift from the Lord. Don't hold back in your grief, but also don't be shy in your gratitude. The next chapter is on hope—we'll explore what hope is, what hope looks like, and why hope is the soul's lifeline. But we have to start here. We have to begin with lifting our eyes.

In her book *The Hiding Place,* Corrie ten Boom tells the moving story of surviving the infamous Nazi death camps. When Corrie and her sister, Betsie, were moved to a barrack that was crawling with fleas, Betsie discovered the key to contentment in 1 Thessalonians, "Rejoice always, pray without ceasing, give thanks in all circumstances" (1 Thess. 5:16–18). And so the sisters began to praise the Lord for the fact that they were together, for their Bible, for other prisoners who could hear the gospel. Then, Betsie did something almost unthinkable: she thanked God for the fleas. The fleas were a nuisance but came with an unexpected blessing because the guards avoided searching their barracks for fear of becoming infested themselves. The women were able to have Bible studies in the barracks with a great deal of freedom. God used fleas to protect the women from abuse and harassment and enabled desperate women to hear the comforting, hope-giving Word of God.[10]

Even though it's not always our first reaction, thankfulness in all circumstances is indeed possible! As we've seen from the biblical and contemporary examples in this chapter, thankfulness and joy are deeply intentional attitudes, rather than fleeting feelings.

Praise the Lord

Even though you might not feel like it, begin praising God right where you are. This act will begin to reorient your heart. By allowing your wounds to propel you in worship, you'll continue to go deeper in your relationship with the Lord.

INVOLVE YOUR COMMUNITY

I urge you to take care of yourself throughout this grieving process. If you're unable to care for yourself or your family, ask for help from a family member, friend, or your church. Asking for help can be difficult, but sometimes it's necessary. You'd be amazed at the number of people who really do want to help, but don't know how. Don't be afraid to tell them exactly what you need. Be open with your family and friends about what you're going through even if it feels difficult and uncomfortable. Sharing your story will allow your community to participate in and empathize with your struggles.

While I am encouraging openness, this doesn't mean

that you have to share your struggles with everyone in your life. Some things are better shared within a close, trusted group. Begin sharing with a few of the people closest to you who know how to encourage you best. The Lord may call you to share more widely one day, but don't feel like you have to tell everyone who asks all the details of your situation. The more widely you share, the more you're opening yourself up to unwelcome opinions. It's wise to draw some boundaries.

When a church responds with compassion and empathy, it can be a powerful resource. If you aren't a part of a local church, put down this book, and go find one right now. It's of utmost importance to be in a community of believers who know you, your heart, and your struggles. Talk about this trial with your pastor, an elder, or a support group. Since the longing for children isn't limited to married couples, I think churches should strive to create open and safe places for *all* people to share their desire for children. Many single women have a great longing for children. It can be easy for the church to overlook singles in this context, because actually having children feels so far removed from their current circumstance.

My friend Melady is one of the most gorgeous and tenderhearted women I've ever met. She's in her midforties, single, and barren. I chatted with her about her journey, and she shared these encouraging words:

In my times of grief, I had the tendency to withdraw and isolate myself. My recommendation would be to fight the temptation to do that. Scripture teaches us to encourage one another and build one another up (1 Thess. 5:11), so I would encourage those walking this journey to pray and ask the Lord to bring someone across your path who is enduring the same struggle or in some way can relate to your pain. You may think that no one understands, but you will be surprised and amazed how He will be faithful to answer your prayer. The support from the body of Christ is very important.

Know Your Limits

Personally, I have decided I can't go to every baby shower to which I'm invited. It's simply too painful. There's a fine line between rejoicing with those who rejoice and walking into a situation you know is going to take you to a trying place. I typically only attend baby showers for my very closest friends—even then, it's extremely difficult, and I usually go home in tears. Figure out what you can and can't handle and don't feel pressured to explain yourself to others. Make sure you're getting enough rest and sufficient space and time to process.

The next step of the journey is toward hope. Is your heart ready for some refreshment and some encouragement? Let's go!

REFLECTION & DISCUSSION

How does it make you feel knowing there are women in the Bible who struggled with childlessness?

What are some of the myths about grieving that you've believed?

How can you cultivate gratitude, even in the midst of trials?

What are some ways that you can involve your community as you grieve?

How do you see God's grace and love in this chapter?

FIVE

WE HAVE THIS HOPE!
What Does Real Hope Look Like?

*T*oday I have the privilege of working on child welfare policy on Capitol Hill in Washington, D.C., a job I never expected I'd have. In 2013, I moved to D.C. after God derailed my original plans. I first started working at a nonprofit and was wondering what I was doing in this strange city.

At Liberty, I studied International Relations and had been planning on moving overseas after I graduated. I knew I couldn't have my own children and was still wrestling through a lot of grief, but I also had a strong desire to care for orphans and vulnerable children. Since adoption has been such an integral part of my life, I wanted to make a difference in the lives of other children who, like me, came from difficult backgrounds. The clearest way I knew to do this was to move overseas and work as a missionary at an orphanage. In my mind, I had glamorized missions, and I had dreams of being the next Mother Teresa.

God knew the pride that was in my heart, and instead of allowing me to move overseas, He directed my path to the nation's capital. While I enjoyed my work at the nonprofit, I felt out of place. I wanted to be helping children in some capacity, but God wasn't making that dream a reality. Since my personal passions weren't lining up with my professional work, I decided to begin volunteering at the local pregnancy center. There, I had the honor of walking with women through difficult life situations. I loved getting to play a small role in making a difference in the lives of these women and children as time passed and I settled into life in D.C.

I had friends who worked in government jobs on the Hill, and they would ask me if I ever considered a similar career. The allure of working on Capitol Hill never appealed to me that much, but I would reply, "If I did consider it, there's only one person I'd want to work for." The congressman to whom I was referring had written and passed the most pro-life pieces of legislation and was the co-chair of the Adoption Caucus, the Foster Youth Caucus, and the Orphans and Vulnerable Children Caucus. His heart for children greatly appealed to me. He was one out of 535 members of Congress, and I never thought I'd have the chance to work for him.

Until one day, a friend of mine sent me the link to a job opening in his office, and I applied. I was offered the job! I saw no obvious reason why they should hire me—I had no previous Hill experience and my qualifications weren't outstanding, but I jumped in with both feet, ready to learn.

Looking back, I can see the Lord's hand in directing my path to D.C. He knew I needed to be humbled and ordained many events to rid me of my pride and teach me to rely on Him. Having the opportunity to work on policies to make the lives of other vulnerable children easier is one of the greatest privileges of my life. Policy matters, and I've learned new skills and gained knowledge that I never would have gotten if I'd immediately moved overseas.

As I write this chapter, it's chilly and rainy in Washington, D.C. I am feeling irritable and grumpy, and the last thing I feel like doing is digging even deeper into my own pain. But also, Sunday is Mother's Day. I truly believe there are many who need this message of hope and healing, but tonight, I don't feel like being the one to write these words. I sense the Lord prompting me to spend time with Him. I'm not proud of my response: "Lord, don't You know I have a deadline? I don't have time to spend time with You." Whoops! As soon as I hear those words leave my mouth, I am convicted of my arrogant and self-centered attitude. I break down and weep, questioning whether I can write this book and asking God why He called me to do this.

I share this so you understand that I still have difficult days. Even though I still get frustrated over the fact that this trial still hurts, it's a realistic picture of our need for hope that will sustain us in moments of sorrow, pain, and doubt. In the midst of grieving our dream of motherhood, it is vital for our soul's survival that we fix our eyes on God. As believers in Jesus Christ, we have the key to a supernatural hope: "We have this hope as an anchor for the soul, firm and secure" (Heb. 6:19 NIV).

The author of Hebrews uses a metaphor here that's used often throughout the Scriptures: a boat at sea. When faced with storms big or small, a sailor can drop his anchor beneath the waves to keep the boat secured to a particular spot. Anchors are what keep sailors from drifting and crashing into the rocks, destroying their ships, and taking their lives. When the storms of life overwhelm and threaten to undo us, we need an anchor tethering us to safety or else we'd certainly be lost. If Jesus is the anchor, then hope is the lifeline for our souls.

As the weeks turned into months, I found myself facing a question, "What was the anchor of my faith in the waves of the storm of childlessness?" I wanted to want Jesus to be my anchor, but choosing Him as my anchor hasn't always been my default. It was easier for me, instead, to choose external people and places as my anchor. I began sharing my childlessness with a select few, but once I did, I expected way too much out of them. I wanted them to anchor my faith, and while having friends is vital during trials, they can't be our anchors.

WHERE DOES HOPE COME FROM?

In college, I took a class on the book of Romans. Typically these types of classes were filled with biblical studies students, but I'd heard nothing but incredible things about the class, and I had a free slot in my schedule, so I signed up. Little did I know that this class would not only change the way I study and read my Bible, it would teach me in deep and profound ways what salvation meant. Not that we can ever fully grasp what Jesus did for us when He bore our sin upon Himself, but as I went chapter by chapter through Romans, I fell so in love with the Lord, with theology, and with the concepts of justification, sanctification, and glorification.

I enrolled in the class three years after I found out about my childlessness. In addition to falling more in love with Christ in that precious class, I also began to learn what hope really is. A wonderful description comes from Romans 5:1–4 (NIV).

> Therefore, since we have been justified through faith, we have peace with God through our Lord Jesus Christ, through whom we have gained access by faith into this grace in which we now stand. And we boast in the hope of the glory of God. Not only so, but we also glory in our sufferings, because we know that suffering produces perseverance; perseverance, character; and character, hope.

Hope comes from God, but it's not the first thing that follows suffering. The Lord knows that oftentimes, our hearts need to be trained so that whenever hope comes, we'll see it for what it really is. Because hope looks different than we imagine, we need to experience perseverance, and from perseverance, character.

According to the Merriam-Webster's dictionary, the definition of hope is "to desire with expectation of fulfillment" or "to expect with confidence."[1] We can pray with Paul, "may the God of hope fill you with all joy and peace in believing, so that by the power of the Holy Spirit you may abound in hope" (Rom. 15:13). We have the capacity to walk forward with hope and joy, even in the face of disappointment or tragedy.

Our hearts must be trained to hope against all odds, even in the midst of difficulty. As you begin healing, take note of how the Lord is changing and shaping you. I can look back and see how I've grown since that fateful November day. I'm a softer, tenderer woman. I'm more resilient and joyful. But perhaps the most important thing that's changed about me as a result of my suffering is that I can more clearly see the ways the Lord has been faithful. When you're on the hunt for those glimpses of His faithfulness, you recognize them all the time.

Hope is impossible unless we keep our eyes fixed on the Lord. We can hope *for* a number of different things, but we need real, lasting hope to sustain us even if the Lord never gives us what we desire.

WHAT IS REAL HOPE?

It can be so easy to place our hope in a longed-for baby. Motherhood becomes the condition for all our future joy and happiness. When we are disappointed in that, we don't want to continue hoping. It feels too hard; it hurts too much. So, how do we regain hope? How do we join the rank of the saints who were not overcome by the trials and challenges they faced? How do we display a hope like Job, who refused the suggestion of his wife to "curse God and die"? How do we walk through seasons of sorrow, through childless days and years, and refuse to give up our hope?

First, I think it's helpful to distinguish between

worldly hope and the faith-filled, supernatural hope God provides. When the world hopes, it's not truly anchored to anything. And it is often self-serving. Worldly hope is more of a wish than an actual, deeply rooted hope. Theologian R. C. Sproul says, "Hope is not simply a wish . . . rather, it is that which latches on to the certainty of the promises of the future that God has made."[2]

Common statements that exhibit our temporal, worldly hope are:

I hope it's sunny tomorrow.

I hope I find a parking spot at the grocery store.

I hope my friends remember my birthday.

I hope my husband makes dinner.

I hope I'm on time to my meeting.

While those aren't bad things per se, we have to see them for what they are: wishes for temporary pleasures or benefits. It's perfectly natural to wish to get pregnant or wish to be a mother. However, we must recognize that those outcomes won't in themselves truly satisfy our souls. When discussing the hope that will surely last—our eternal, sustaining hope—it's helpful to substitute the word "hope" with the word "know." This exercise helps me ensure that I'm not hoping in something temporal, but that my hope is deeply rooted in what I know to be true of God. We can certainly wish for certain things, but it can easily set us up for failure if we don't get them. When we place our hope in what we know to be true, we give our Father the freedom to fill in our story as He sees fit.

The following statements include the clear but unspoken hope that flows from our faith in Christ:

I know the Lord will be faithful.

I know this trial isn't the end of my story.

I know the Lord loves me.

I know the Lord won't forsake me, even in my hardest season.

I know the Lord sees me when I cry.

HOPE IN GOD BUILDS TRUST IN HIM

Disappointment occurs when worldly hope and godly hope are confused. It's easy to get the two mixed up. We can know that we are anchored to real hope when it aligns with the promises of Scripture and the character of God. This hope is rooted in God, and because God never changes, neither will our source of hope. As time passes, our level of hope grows, because we learn that the Lord is trustworthy. Learning to hope is like learning to walk. The first few steps a child takes are shaky and unsure. Our Father, with His open arms, seems so far away. But each step teaches us that when we fall, God will be right there to catch us. We can trust in our Father's love and care.

HOPE ISN'T STRAIGHTFORWARD

The journey toward hope and healing won't necessarily be straightforward or clear. The road will get rocky and uneven, sometimes you may even lose your way. This process may be messy, dark, and mysterious. And your path to healing will likely look very different from that of others. There's no one-size-fits-all journey toward wholeness. The most important thing is that you get there, and I assure you, you will get there! We shouldn't think of hope as a linear path. I used to believe that I had already walked through my grief and pain, walked toward hope and healing, and moved on with the rest of my life.

It's true that the further away you get from a loss, the easier it becomes, and the more perspective you gain. But the journey is not necessarily a sequential one. I've been shocked to discover that I can have hope in the midst of my pain instead of on the other side of my pain. Hope and grief can coexist, they aren't at odds with each other. Hope is the reminder that there's something better out there. Even if the only hope we have at times is the hope of heaven that propels our heart forward.

HOPE IS A CHOICE

The winter after my diagnosis was hard. My heart felt as cold as the weather, and hope was the furthest thing from my mind. I didn't feel like being hopeful, in fact, I felt quite the opposite. My heart quickly tumbled into despair, and I remained there for a long time. But as I wallowed in my pain, hurt, and bitterness, I realized that I wasn't getting any better. The grieving process is incredibly important, but I wasn't in any kind of process. I was stuck. I was lying motionless in my sorrow. Nothing was propelling me forward. Eventually I decided I didn't want to live like that. Barrenness will always be part of my story, but I had to make a choice: was I going to let my circumstances control my life, or was I going to begin to live wholeheartedly and hopefully in the midst of my sorrow?

The journey toward hope often begins with desperation. May we take our cue from David, who did not hold back in pouring out his heart to God: "I waited patiently for the LORD; he inclined to me and heard my cry. He drew me up from the pit of destruction, out of the miry bog, and set my feet upon a rock, making my steps secure. He put a new song in my mouth, a song of praise to our God. Many will see and fear, and put their trust in the LORD" (Ps. 40:1–3). It can be so easy to allow your pain to overshadow everything in your life, but it is possible to choose hope.

In his book *Spiritual Depression*, D. Martyn Lloyd-Jones discusses the importance of talking to your soul and of instructing your soul toward hope and toward healing. In fact, he said that the main art in the matter of spiritual living is knowing how to handle yourself. The psalmists give us an excellent example of what this looks like, and we can echo their words, "Why are you downcast, O my soul?" Lloyd-Jones instructs us on how to handle our souls and says that we should remind ourselves to "hope in God" instead of muttering in a "depressed, unhappy way." But we can't stop there. He says we must go on to remind ourselves "who God is, and what God is and what God has done, and what God has pledged Himself to do. Then having done that, end on this great note: defy yourself, and defy other people, and defy the devil and the whole world, and say with this man: 'I shall yet praise Him for the help of His countenance, who is also the health of my countenance and my God.'"[3]

Throughout the Bible, and throughout the ages, Christians have had to remind themselves of things they know to be true. There's a reason we're so often compared to sheep in the Bible: we're restless creatures, prone to wander, and with a great need for a shepherd.[4] We desperately need the Lord walking before us, beside us, and behind us, shepherding our hearts and our lives. In Psalms 42 and 43, we see the psalmist talking to himself and to his soul. The writer is reminding his soul that ours is a living God (42:2), He is present with us day and night (42:8), that we are to bless the Lord and remember His faithfulness (42:5), and that we are to rest and hope in God (43:5).

Learn to talk *to* your soul, instead of automatically accepting every emotion and every feeling that comes your way. A practical way to do this when you're feeling depressed or sorrowful is to pause and talk to yourself. I often try to find a quiet place where I can be alone and say aloud, "Chelsea, you're feeling a lot of things right now, and it's completely okay to feel them. However, you can't stay in these feelings forever. What can you do in this moment to take steps toward hope?" I'll then spend time reciting some of God's promises.

I've had to remind myself that my feelings aren't bad, but they can't be my guiding light. Hope isn't a fluffy feeling. If we always felt like hoping, there'd be no need for this chapter. Biblical truth should inform our feelings, and hope should be the thing we strive for. May our emotions submit to God's promises and truth. As you do this, cling to and pray these words: "On the day I called, you answered me; my strength of soul you increased. . . . Though I walk in the midst of trouble, you preserve my life" (Ps. 138: 3, 7).

The book of Lamentations is perhaps the most sorrowful book of the Bible, written to "express grief over the fall of Jerusalem and confidence in the faithfulness of God."[5] In the second half of the book, we read, "But this I call to mind, and therefore I have hope" (Lam. 3:21). From there, Jeremiah talks about the steadfast love of the Lord, God's mercies, hoping in the Lord, and waiting upon the Lord. Jeremiah is teaching us a lesson we've begun to learn as we've worked our way through this book. He's teaching us how to fix our eyes on the Lord.

What things do we need to call to mind to give our hearts hope? Our hearts desperately need to be reminded of the things we know to be true, truths that won't change and won't disappoint us, and that will last for eternity. We are sometimes disappointed by the Lord's plans, but often that's because—with hearts tainted by a fallen world—we've misplaced our hope all along. If our hope was truly in the Lord, we wouldn't be quite as angry when we don't get what we desire.

Words from the well-known and well-loved hymn "It Is Well with My Soul" have been sung for years and have brought comfort and hope to thousands of people. But few realize those same words were penned following tragedy. Horatio Spafford lost all four of his daughters in one day, after he had already lost his young son to illness. Two years after the great Chicago fire almost ruined Spafford, he bid his daughters and his wife farewell as they set sail for a trip to England. But their ship was hit by another vessel and all four daughters were killed. His wife survived and sent him a telegram when she arrived that read, "Saved alone." Spafford left right away to be with his grieving wife, and en route to England, he penned the powerful words to the hymn, "It Is Well with My Soul."[6]

I'm sure you're familiar with the lyrics, but if not, I encourage you to look them up or listen to the song. I find the first two stanzas particularly meaningful in my journey through childlessness.

> *When peace, like a river, attendeth my way,*
> *When sorrows like sea billows roll;*
> *Whatever my lot, Thou hast taught me to say,*
> *It is well, it is well with my soul.*
> *It is well with my soul,*
> *It is well, it is well with my soul.*

> *Though Satan should buffet, though trials should come,*
> *Let this blest assurance control,*
> *That Christ hath regarded my helpless estate,*
> *And hath shed His own blood for my soul.*
> *It is well with my soul,*
> *It is well, it is well with my soul.*

Pastor and preacher John Piper has described Spafford's ability to hope, even in the midst of extreme loss, this way: "He knew Christ loved him. He saw it in the cross. And when he gets to the end [of the song], he has Christ coming back with a great triumph not to judge him but to save him and to raise his daughters from the dead so 'it is well with my soul.' The great question is how could it be well?"[7]

Oftentimes, we don't like the answer. God has a purpose in our pain, but it's frustrating that we may never understand why the Lord allows something into our lives. Many times, trials and sorrows are what the Lord uses to shape us into His character and likeness. In our limited understanding of the kingdom of heaven, this is never the way we would have chosen to grow. We have an aversion to pain and try to craft our lives to avoid it at all costs. The true hope of a Christian is eternity spent with our heavenly Father, and that is absolutely guaranteed to us.

I love when I'm able to see spiritual truths like this in everyday things. Gardening has been a place where I've learned many lessons. Growing up, gardening was a big part of my childhood, and I loved harvesting fresh vegetables and picking flowers to freshen up the house. What I didn't like was weeding the garden. It was hard, painful, time consuming, and annoying. But that work has to be done just as it has to be done in our lives, so that the seeds we plant—seeds of love, seeds of faith, seeds pointing people to Christ—can grow and mature, especially through difficult seasons. And seeds take time to grow.

We live in an instant gratification culture where we get frustrated if we have to wait too long for anything, much less the deepest desires of our heart. Throughout Scripture, we're reminded to "wait for the LORD; be strong, and let you heart take courage; wait for the LORD!" (Ps. 27:14). Waiting goes against our human nature, but it's possible to wait and to grow in character, even through our pain: "We rejoice in our sufferings, knowing that suffering produces endurance, and endurance produces character, and character produces hope, and hope does not put us to shame, because God's love has been poured into our hearts through the Holy Spirit who has been given to us" (Rom. 5:3–5).

By walking through trials, we change. Our hearts gain strength and endurance, we lean into God in ways we probably wouldn't if it weren't for our trials. Through the difficulties, the Lord refines our character. He prunes the parts of us that don't look like Him. We probably won't even realize what's happening in the process, but we're becoming more like our Savior. If we're pressing hard into Jesus through our childlessness, we'll inevitably become more like Him. And as our character grows, hope will be produced. Beloved, don't allow your heart to be choked out by bitterness. It's a temptation in the midst of sorrow. Instead, allow the Lord's tender care to soften your heart, and love out of the abundance of that.

One of the most influential people on my life has been author C. S. Lewis. I've eagerly read his Chronicles of Narnia and soaked up his wisdom, but it is an excerpt from his book *The Four Loves* that has challenged me to have a right heart, even in the most difficult circumstances.

There is no safe investment. To love at all is to be vulnerable. Love anything, and your heart will certainly be wrung and possibly be broken. If you want to make sure of keeping it intact, you must give your heart to no one, not even to an animal. Wrap it carefully round with hobbies and little luxuries; avoid all entanglements; lock it up safe in the casket or coffin of your selfishness. But in that casket—safe, dark, motionless, airless—it will change. It will not be broken; it will become unbreakable, impenetrable, irredeemable. The only place outside Heaven where you can be perfectly safe from all the dangers and perturbations of love is Hell.[8]

By remaining tenderhearted in difficult and painful

times, your life will point to the work of Christ in you. Hold on to the truth that the Lord is faithful, and hold on to the hope of His steadfast love for you, no matter how your story ends. Lift your eyes to the Lord and say with the psalmist, "Why are you cast down, O my soul, and why are you in turmoil within me? Hope in God; for I shall again praise him, my salvation and my God" (Ps. 43:5). Hope will come.

REFLECTION & DISCUSSION

Are you tempted to look in the wrong places or to the wrong people for hope?

How can you remind yourself of the things you know to be true (e.g., God's promises, God's character, the hope God offers)?

How can you live in the tension of sorrow and hope coexisting?

How do you see God's grace and love in this chapter?

SIX

WAYS TO LIVE
OUT THE LONGING

How You Can
Still Be a Mother

W hile your path to motherhood might look different than you originally thought it would, there
are many incredibly beautiful, Christ-centered ways to
fulfill your heart's desire. As I have discovered through
my work on child welfare policy on Capitol Hill, it is
possible to serve in a "mothering" role without conceiving your own biological children, and there are many opportunities in our world to nurture and care for children.
I encourage you to read this chapter prayerfully as you
consider how the Lord might be calling you to love and
serve. For surely this instruction applies to all of us:

You shall teach [God's words] to your children,
talking of them when you are sitting in your house,
and when you are walking by the way, and when
you lie down, and when you rise. (Deut. 11:19)

The Lord promises to give wisdom to those who lack
it (James 1:5). He'll be with you and equip you as you
begin praying and seeking. Your longing to be a mother
doesn't have to be in vain!

BECOME A SPIRITUAL MOTHER

One way to fulfill your desire to be a mother is to look for
opportunities to minister, to mentor, or to care for children. Even if you're childless, you can still nurture and
minister to others, children included. In fact, I've found
that getting involved in ministry is an effective way to
take my eyes off my own struggle. Perhaps you could
teach Sunday school at your church, serve in the nursery
or youth group, volunteer as a mentor, or tutor at a local
school. I guarantee there are many children around you
who need a godly influence in their lives.

When I moved to D.C., I befriended a young woman
who was only a few years younger than I was. I quickly
learned that she'd miscarried multiple times and was
pregnant again. Eventually, I got to know her younger
siblings, who would hug my neck every time I saw them.
My relationship with this young mother blossomed into
a mentorship, and to her siblings, I became Aunt Chelsea. I never dreamed what an impact this would have on
me. I'd set out to help others, but instead found myself

being ministered to. My heart was aching to be a mother, and while I wasn't a mother to my own children, it was so special to take on the role of mentor and honorary aunt to precious people in my community.

BECOME MORE THAN A RELATIVE

The role of an aunt is one that's often overlooked and undervalued. If you have siblings with children, you can have a powerful influence in the lives of your nieces and nephews. Bible teacher Kelly Minter explains the importance of her role as an aunt: "As a single woman, or any woman who has a void in her life, we can focus solely on what we're missing, or we can claim the place God has given us with our nieces and nephews, a place no one else has."[1]

Begin thinking of ways to intentionally pour into their lives and look for opportunities to speak truth to them. They'll feel special when you are creative in planning ways to love and care for them so you can build a unique relationship with them. Perhaps you can take your niece or nephew for a weekly outing, babysit occasionally, or invite them to spend a weekend at your house. My mom has one sister who was frequently at our home. Her presence was a vital part of my formative years, because I knew I had the unconditional love of another adult woman.

Spiritual mentoring, whether that comes from our mothers or other women in our lives, can be invaluable. Multiple times throughout the book of Proverbs, Solomon reminds his readers not to forsake their mother's teaching. The famous thirty-first chapter of Proverbs is written about the characteristics of a godly woman. All women have the ability to seek after godliness and use their life experience to love and shepherd another person in the faith.

If you aren't sure how to fill the role of spiritual mother, look to people in your life or your church who already model this well for you. Who have been some of the most influential women in your life? What are the specific things you admire about them? Maybe you have been profoundly nurtured by your own mother, or maybe it's been an aunt, grandma, or another woman who chose to walk alongside you as a mentor or friend. Love knows no boundaries; when someone loves you and truly cares about your well-being, it doesn't matter if you're related to them or not.

There have been several women a few steps beyond me on life's path who have loved me and invested in me in addition to my mother. I look up to them and respect their walks with the Lord, their relationships with their husbands, and how they handle and construct their lives. I aspire to follow their godly example. Beatrice is one of those women for me. Her heart is full of love, and her tongue is always ready to impart wisdom from her long life. Even though I don't see her nearly as often as I'd like, every time we do spend time together, we comfortably slip right back into sharing our hearts. Recently, I had to go home to North Carolina for a major surgery that required two weeks of bed rest. Seeing my dear friend before my surgery was important to me, so I traveled home early to make time to visit.

We went out for lunch on a warm July afternoon. She asked lots of questions as we caught up. "You know, Chelsea," she said, "as you've shared stories of Michael, living and working in D.C., writing, and your friendships, all I can keep thinking about is how God has His hand in every detail of your life." She went on to encourage me with things she'd seen the Lord do in and through me. The love and support she's given have been invaluable. I want to be that kind of woman.

Whether you are discipling a high school or college student, mentoring a child with no godly models, or relishing your role as an aunt, you can be a spiritual mother. This is an endeavor just as worthy and noble as having your own children, and it's a way to exercise your nurturing spirit.

Learn to ask good questions of those you choose to mentor. Asking questions draws someone out and helps them articulate what they are thinking and feeling. I have found that a few helpful questions to regularly ask include:

- What challenges are you currently facing?
- In what specific ways do you see the Lord working in your life?
- How can I love and serve you?
- What are some things you're thankful for?
- How do you sense God's care for you?
- How can I pray for you?

One word of caution though. Don't try to fill the void in your life with spiritual children until you've worked through your own pain and have come to some sense of peace with your childlessness. If you rush too quickly into mentoring or discipleship before you're ready, there's a risk you will seek to fulfill your unmet expectations and desires in that relationship.

How can you avoid this? Make sure to surround yourself with people who aren't afraid to tell you the truth about yourself and your circumstances. Ask your pastor or others who know your level of spiritual maturity if you're in a place that you can handle it. If you begin to walk down this road and realize that it's too much to handle right now, push pause to allow your heart to continue healing. (Be honest with your mentee and help direct them to another mentor.) As we discussed in the previous chapter, don't set expectations on a healing process for yourself. There's no one you're accountable to except the Lord, and there's no rush to become a spiritual mother.

BECOME AN ADOPTIVE PARENT

There may be no better illustration of the gospel than adoption. Think about your own spiritual adoption. You were hopeless, wretched, forsaken, and headed for destruction. Yet the Lord stepped into your story, rescued you, redeemed you, and called you His child: "For you did not receive the spirit of slavery to fall back into fear, but you have received the Spirit of adoption as sons, by whom we cry, 'Abba! Father!'" (Rom. 8:15). Is anything more beautiful and stunning than that? Few topics excite me more than the topic of adoption. Because it's in integral part of my story and because I'm a Christian, I know I've been doubly adopted! A large part of my love stems from my personal connection with adoption. If Bobby and Christie Patterson hadn't made the decision to travel to Romania and choose me, I shudder to think what kind of life I would have had. My siblings and I grew up knowing that we were intentionally sought out, chosen, and loved.

There is a great need for caring and loving people to enter into the lives of orphans and vulnerable children around the world. Currently, there are approximately 140 million orphaned children worldwide.[2] It's important to note that this doesn't necessarily mean both parents are deceased. In some of these cases, like my own birth and adoption story, the parents are unable to take care of their child and there is no other family member to whom they can turn, thereby, "orphaning" the child. World Orphans, a nonprofit with the mission of "empowering the church to care for orphans until they all have homes" published an article with the heartbreaking statistic that "more than 800 million people are living on less than $1.25 per day, making poverty the leading cause of family disruption."[3]

Children thrive best in families, not institutions or orphanages, so every effort should be made by governments and nongovernmental organizations (NGOs) to equip families to stay together. Unfortunately, that isn't always possible, and many children are in need of safe, permanent, and loving families. Due to the unknowns in both the process and outcome, adoption can feel overwhelming and scary for a couple that has already been through the pain of childlessness.

To take a first step in combatting those fears, some of which are unfounded, let's look at a few misconceptions about the adoption process.

Adoption Is Too Expensive

Many couples say they would love to adopt, but they don't have the money. While adoption can be incredibly expensive, especially international adoption, it doesn't have to be. An international adoption can cost more than $40,000 because many countries require prospective parents to visit the child before they are allowed to legally adopt.[4] Then, they have to take another trip to that country to finalize the adoption. International court, legal, and adoption fees add up all too quickly. Domestic adoption can be less expensive depending on whether it is handled independently or through an agency, while adopting through the foster care system is virtually free.[5] Many organizations provide financial assistance for adoptive parents. (See the additional resources at the end of this book.)

Another option to consider when looking at the financial responsibility of adoption is your local church. Many churches have benevolence funds for people with specific needs, and I know of several churches that have funds designated for adoptive couples. Tell your pastor if you're interested in adoption. You never know what's available through your local church or denomination.

If finances are the primary reason you're not considering adoption, I urge you to reconsider. My parents adopted six children on my father's salary. It was important to my parents that my mom have the ability to stay home and raise the children. I've never seen anyone work harder than my dad. After he'd tuck us in at night, I knew he'd often return to his work for a few hours. His mission was to provide for his family. While my family isn't wealthy by any stretch of the imagination, we're truly rich in love. My parents have told me that they could have chosen to have a large bank account and live an extremely comfortable life, but they chose to invest in something that will outlast and outlive them: their children. They made investments in eternity.

Adoption Is Just Too Difficult

While I don't want to paint adoption as a process filled with ease and bliss, I believe the blessing is well worth the challenges. The need for adoption is a result of the fall. God's original design for families was for one man and one woman to be fruitful and to fill the earth with children. When sin entered the world, everything felt the effects of it, including families. Adoption always begins with loss. A child has been abandoned by or separated from her parents and placed in the arms of another family or an orphanage director. Even if a child is adopted at a younger age, that life begins out of brokenness and loss. When an adoption is finalized, there's redemption because of the act of adoption, but the child has still experienced trauma.

Adoptive parents need to be ready to handle the challenges born out of that trauma. When potential adoptive parents are going through the adoption process, they are required to attend classes that teach them how to care for an adopted child and the particular needs that child has developed as a result of his experience. Now more than ever, an abundance of resources are available to inform and equip potential adoptive parents and help ensure a successful adoption. Read good books on adoption. Talk to people who have walked the road before you. Remember that just because something is difficult doesn't mean we shouldn't do it!

I Can't Love an Adopted Child Like I Would Love My Own

If I talk long enough to people about adoption, inevitably they raise this concern. This breaks my heart every time I hear it. If we have accepted God's adoption of us, and if we desire to live out the gospel message, this misconception shouldn't deter us. God chose us when we didn't deserve it, and there was nothing lovely about us. As John Piper says, "The gospel is not a picture of adoption; adoption is a picture of the gospel."[6]

When I was first dating Michael, he told me in a tear-filled conversation that he needed some time to process what adoption would mean for him and for our future life if we decided to continue moving forward in our relationship. After what felt like forever to me (though it was just a few weeks), we circled back on this particular discussion. He shared that he'd never expected to be faced with choosing adoption so early on in a relationship. Like many of us, he had assumed he'd someday have his own children. As he shared his heart, I cried, knowing that I'd never be able to give him children and scared that he would tell me adoption wasn't for him. Instead, his words were tender and encouraging, "Sweetheart, as I've been wrestling and praying over the past few weeks, I've realized that the most important thing isn't having a child that looks like me. The most important thing is raising a child to look like Christ."

I've had the privilege of chatting with hundreds of people who have adopted. Countless couples have told me that as soon as the child was placed in their arms as their legal child, it didn't matter to them whether or not it was their "own" child; what mattered was in a single moment, they became parents.

I recognize that not everyone is called to adoption or to being a foster parent, but we are all called to care for the orphan. James 1:27 (NIV) tells us that the "religion that

God our Father accepts as pure and blameless is this: to look after orphans and widows in their distress and to keep oneself from being polluted by the world." What is James telling us? He's instructing us to pay attention and care for the most vulnerable people.

My favorite translations of this verse use the word "fatherless" instead of "orphan." Many of the children we consider to be orphans have at least one living parent who's simply unable to properly care for them. Maybe you're not in a position to adopt, or maybe you don't feel called to adoption. But I invite you to get involved in caring for children.

BECOME AN ADVOCATE

The best advocacy is inspired by personal experience. Because I have firsthand experience with adoption, my passion informs my professional work on Capitol Hill, where I advocate for child welfare policy. Many people may feel intimidated by advocacy work, but your desire to care for children can be a catalyst for being a voice for the voiceless. You don't have to work on Capitol Hill to advocate for children. There are many ways to help:

Pray

Never underestimate the power of prayer! Petition the heart of our Father on behalf of vulnerable children. Ask the Lord to provide safe, permanent, and loving homes and families. Pray for the families that adopt children. Ultimately, pray that the souls of orphans and vulnerable children would be drawn to Christ.

Give

Another way you can help is to financially support those who are called to adopt. As we've discussed, one hurdle people have to overcome regarding adoption is adequate financial resources. Consider contributing financially to a couple or family that desires to adopt. Many are willing to open their hearts and homes but don't have sufficient means to cover the costs. You'll never regret investing in helping them accomplish this. Proverbs 19:17 encourages us in this: "Whoever is generous to the poor lends to the LORD, and he will repay him for his deed."

Get Involved

My work on child welfare policy has led me to meet some of the most passionate advocates for adoption and vulnerable children. While many of the people I interact with have a personal connection to child welfare, not all do. Recently, I was meeting with a gentleman on a particular policy concern he had. Earlier in his life, he'd been a successful lawyer, and today he spends his time doing pro bono work for children. Near the end of the meeting, I asked him why he chose to spend the later years of his life helping children. He said that there used to be a time when people did the right thing simply because it was the right thing to do, and caring for children is the right thing to do.

Each of us can use our voice to advocate on behalf of fatherless, vulnerable, abused, or marginalized children. Get involved in your local community as a court-appointed child advocate or ask your pastor to preach about God's command to care for them. The Lord has entrusted each one of us with different gifts, resources, and schedules. Consider big and small ways you can be a voice for children.

You can be part of building a strong community that's dedicated to loving and supporting adoptive families and those involved in adoption and foster care. There are many practical ways to serve these folks, such as babysitting or funding an occasional date night, providing a meal, asking sincerely how they're doing and taking the time to listen to the answer, or mentoring a foster or adopted child.

BECOME A PARENT
THROUGH MEDICAL INTERVENTION

This is a complex topic that extends beyond our discussion of alternative ways to live out a parental or nurturing role, but I feel these options still need to be mentioned, especially since they may be relevant to many readers.

Conception through In Vitro Fertilization (IVF)

Though it's only been around for about forty years, in vitro fertilization (IVF) is becoming a more and more popular option for couples who struggle to conceive.[7] Several million babies worldwide have been born through IVF, which has become a multimillion dollar industry.[8] As Christians, it's extremely important to understand *exactly* what is involved with IVF, a type of assisted reproductive technology (ART). IVF, at its most basic level, is the "process of fertilization by extracting eggs, retrieving a sperm sample, and then manually combining the egg and sperm in a laboratory."[9] The embryo(s) are then transferred to the woman's uterus. IVF is a long and tedious process, involving multiple doctor visits, hormone treatments, and other procedures. Although the success rates of IVF are growing, the chances of successful treatment range between 20–35 percent,[10] and the cost of just one treatment can be as high as $15,000.[11]

While I don't presume to know everything about this issue, I believe the ethics of IVF can get very tricky, very fast. A Pew Research study found that "most Americans think that having an abortion is a moral issue. By contrast, the public is much less likely to see other issues involving human embryos—such as stem cell research or in vitro fertilization—as a matter of morality." For instance, only 12 percent of Americans believe that IVF is morally wrong.[12] There are also potential issues with the way certain clinics advertise their services and success rates.

The hosts of the podcast Reveal, an investigative reporting podcast, once covered these concerns.

Success rates are easy to misunderstand and easy to manipulate. In addition to transferring too many embryos at once, clinics might take on only the easiest cases. They can push patients with low chances for success into other treatments not tracked by the CDC [Centers for Disease Control]. Some clinics choose to advertise pregnancy rates instead of live-birth rates, knowing that miscarriages will inevitably happen. Even when success is measured by live births, the numbers can be deceiving. For the purpose of statistics, it doesn't matter whether babies or mothers suffer health complications before, during, or soon after birth.[13]

After an embryo is placed in a womb, the remaining embryos are often frozen for further use or discarded. Many doctors won't bother beginning an IVF treatment unless a woman has embryos frozen in the event a treatment fails. In a recent estimate, there are approximately 600,000 frozen embryos in fertility clinics across the country.[14] Herein lies the ethical and moral dilemma for Christians. A part of being a pro-life Christian is valuing life at all stages. How we think through and interact with IVF will say something to the world about what we value as precious.

Another popular option in IVF treatments is called Preimplantation Genetic Diagnosis (PGD), which involves testing all the embryos and performing genetic profiling so they only implant the "healthy" embryos. There's absolutely nothing wrong with wanting a healthy baby, but I think we can set ourselves up to miss out on the privilege of raising children who are "less than perfect" in the world's eyes. Another red flag with PGD is that this technique can be used to select one sex over another. I believe PGD comes far too close to creating "designer babies."

We shouldn't strive to have a child at the expense of destroying life. As Christians, we must begin with the presupposition that life begins at conception and that all life has innate value: "For you formed my inward parts; you knitted me together in my mother's womb" (Ps. 139:13). Shane Pruitt, the director of evangelism for the Southern Baptists of Texas Convention and a gifted Bible teacher, reminds us that "lives are still lives, even if they're microscopic."[15] While I can't tell you what to do, I strongly urge you to carefully and prayerfully consider all aspects before proceeding with IVF treatments. Be willing to walk away if you get remotely close to "playing God" with human embryos. Consider the sovereignty of

God and ask yourself whether you believe that extends to your infertility. Some additional questions you need to ask yourself:

- Do we really believe that life begins at conception? What exactly does that mean to us?
- Where will we draw the line in our IVF process?
- Will we tell our future child how they were conceived?
- If we do IVF, will we participate in PGDs, such as attempting to select the sex of our baby, rule out potential birth defects, etc.?

Conception through Surrogacy

Another option many couples consider is surrogacy. I've given this option some thought since *technically* I could have my own children. Even though I was born without a uterus, I do have ovaries and eggs, and I could hire a surrogate mother to carry my child. But the costs can quickly reach $150,000, including agency fees, attorneys' fees, screening and surrogate fees, and medical and insurance costs.[16] In addition to wondering whether I could justify spending this much money pursuing motherhood, if I'm honest with myself, I feel like this falls into the category of taking life into my own hands. May we not get so caught up in pursuing having biological children that we act without wisdom or outside of God's will. Considering the financial investment, I feel better about putting my money toward adoption instead.

Though I don't know what your journey toward motherhood looks like, I do know that the Lord will be with you every step and will remain faithful. As you consider what path is right for you, it's important to discuss your thoughts and feelings with those who know you best and can speak with complete honesty into your life. I'd urge you not to make any rash or emotional decisions. The desire to be a mother can be intoxicating and overpowering at times. Give yourself space and time to think through and pray about what option might be best for you. It's also helpful to remember that everyone in your life might not understand your decision or choice. Motherhood is possible—it might look different than you imagined . . . but be everything God has planned.

REFLECTION & DISCUSSION

If you can't have biological children, are you willing to consider one of these options? Why or why not?

If you are considering a different path toward motherhood, have you talked and prayed it over with people?

What option excites you the most? Scares you the most?

How do you see God's grace and love in this chapter?

SEVEN

DON'T WASTE YOUR CHILDLESSNESS

Use Your Suffering to Serve Others

Years have passed since my diagnosis, and I've begun to heal. I've also found a strong desire in my heart to use my suffering to serve others. I had no idea where to begin, especially since I'd kept my childlessness largely private. During the time I began to consider how to steward my trials, I read *Don't Waste Your Life* by John Piper. It remains one of the most influential books I've ever read. The book is a passionate plea to make your life count for eternity.[1]

Piper explains how everything in life can be used for the glory of God and the good of others. He shares a story about a painting his mother hung above the kitchen sink. On the painting were words from a poem by C. T. Studd that read, "Only one life, 'twill soon be past, only what's done for Christ will last." Piper saw those words multiple times throughout the day, and they shaped his heart with an urgency for making an eternal impact. He went on to start an international ministry, preach, write over fifty books, and teach others how to glorify God.

My heart was lit on fire as I learned from the pages of Piper's book how to yearn for eternity. I resolved to make my life count, and that includes my childlessness. I strongly desire that my actions on earth will withstand the test of eternity. Even though I never would have chosen childlessness for myself, I'm now faced with a choice I do control: "What will I do with my suffering?" Childlessness changed me. I began to realize that even though I couldn't change my circumstances, there were things I was in control of—my attitude and my actions. Over the years, I've striven to learn how I could use my childlessness to glorify the Lord and to help others. As I've learned those lessons, I've realized that this perspective is key to experiencing fulfillment in the midst of the struggle.

I'm quick to forget that my actions on earth have eternal consequences. Paul reminds us in 2 Corinthians 4:17–18 that "this light momentary affliction is preparing for us an eternal weight of glory beyond all comparison, as we look not to the things that are seen but to the things that are unseen. For the things that are seen are transient, but the things that are unseen are eternal."

When I first read that verse, I wanted to have a conversation with Paul. It would go something like this, "Paul, my childlessness doesn't feel light and momentary.

It feels heavy and permanent. If I'm honest, it feels more real than eternity does right now."

I imagine Paul being tender in his response as he whispers, "Dear one, I know." He'd probably go on to remind me of the excruciating suffering he'd gone through. "Three times I was beaten with rods. Once I was stoned. Three times I was shipwrecked; a night and a day I was adrift at sea. Chelsea, even though our circumstances are often harder than we'd like, don't lose sight of what God is doing. Fix your eyes on the eternal weight of glory, learn to see the unseen things, the eternal things." I'd walk away from that conversation with a desire to train my eyes to see what God was really up to.

Without first having a desire for the eternal weight of glory, we won't have a desire to use our childlessness. If we don't long for Jesus, how will we long to help others? What is the weight of glory that Paul is describing? My favorite explanation is from the prolific Bible commentary writer Matthew Henry. He described the concept in the following way:

> The apostle and his fellow-sufferers saw their afflictions working towards heaven, and that they would end at last, whereupon they weighed things aright in the balance of the sanctuary; they did as it were put the heavenly glory on one scale and their earthly sufferings on the other; and, pondering things in their thoughts, they found afflictions to be light, and the glory of heaven to be a far more exceeding weight.[2]

Even though it doesn't feel like it now, this momentary pain will pale in comparison to the glory that's waiting for us in heaven.

TRIALS SHAPE OUR CHARACTER

One of the best lessons we can learn as we try to be good stewards of our childlessness is that trials change us. In my suffering, I wanted to know the end result. I wanted to know that it'd all be okay, and that this was just a season. Looking back, I can see God teaching me, growing me, and transforming me. To use a popular but accurate analogy, imagine your life as a tapestry. At the moment, all you can see is the thread, the knots, and the unfinished work. But the Lord is at work, weaving and creating a beautiful masterpiece. Someday when we look back, we'll get glimpses of what the Lord was up to.

In *Walking with God through Pain and Suffering*, Tim Keller reminds us that suffering can refine us rather than destroy us because God Himself walks with us in the fire."[3] My suffering has made me, and continues to make me, more Christlike.

COME AND SEE

The invitation of every Christian life should be "Come and see what God has done" (Ps. 66:5). Opening up our lives, especially in the midst of difficulties, can be challenging, but can serve as a conduit for the work of the Holy Spirit in the life of another person.

One of the first times I witnessed this personally was in college and a few years after my diagnosis. I was a resident assistant responsible for guiding and caring for the young women in my residence hall. Because I went to a Christian university, our weekly hall meetings always included a devotional. One week, as I neared the end of my college career, I decided to share my story and share God's faithfulness. After I opened up and shared the hard things in my life, many of the girls came to me privately to share their hurts and struggles.

So how do we rightly steward both the good things and the hard things the Lord has allowed into our lives? How do we model to the world that Christ is more precious to us than anything else, even the children we long for? The world is watching to see if we'll continue to praise the Lord—even through difficult seasons. How should we respond when we don't get what we want? Remember that your suffering isn't in vain. We may never know the reasons, but we know the God we serve.

DON'T LOSE HEART

Even though we intellectually know that trials are a part of life, when hardship and suffering enter our own story, we're often thrown off guard. Jesus' reminder to His followers was that in the world we "will have tribulation" (John 16:33). We aren't guaranteed an easy life. The beloved twentieth-century author and pastor A. W. Tozer said, "God offers life, but not an improved old life."[4] It's tempting to believe that life will magically get better the moment we choose to follow Christ. However, the opposite is true. The cost of following Christ is death of self, death of our own desires and dreams. However, Jesus tenderly tells us to take heart, because He has overcome the world and He is on our side.

In 2 Corinthians 4:16, right before Paul talks about the eternal weight of glory that's awaiting us in heaven, he exhorts believers: "So we do not lose heart. Though our outer self is wasting away, our inner self is being renewed day by day." This is one of the most countercultural commands I've read. I don't know about you, but when I'm tired or sad, the last thing I feel like doing is continuing to trust. Continuing to hold on to hope can only be done with the Lord's help. It's truly His strength alone that will sustain our hearts through the valleys.

Hopefully, your heart has begun to heal or you are gaining hope that healing is possible. Remember to whom you belong, and remember that the Lord is with you. It's out of the brokenness that redemption comes. Don't let childlessness define you. Even if your circumstances never change, by God's grace *you* will change.

SHARE YOUR STORY IN GOD'S TIME

Sharing your story with others can be a powerful way to utilize your unique experience. When you open up about the deeper, hidden parts of yourself, you invite connection on a more intimate level. When you take the risk to be vulnerable, in effect you are saying, "Me too." You show that you don't have it all together and you are willing to share real life.

Don't feel like you need to begin sharing your story immediately. In fact, it's probably best to give yourself plenty of time and space to process your experience. You don't need to have a formal ministry or share personal details with everyone you meet. Just be aware that someone else might need your story. When you feel you're ready to share it, pray for God to lead you, and begin to intentionally look for opportunities that will allow you to offer support.

One of the most powerful things about sharing your story is allowing people to see how you've honestly struggled with the Lord and to hear you say, "I understand what you're going through. I've been through something similar."

Trials are oftentimes the things the Lord uses the most. In *The Broken Way*, Ann Voskamp writes, "This is how you live with your one broken heart; you give it away."[5]

How does your unique experience of childlessness become a powerful story you can "give away" to encourage others?

BUILD FRIENDSHIPS WITH THE CHILDLESS

A selfless but still fulfilling way to give of yourself during this season is to build intentional friendships with other childless women. Whether they are single women longing for marriage and motherhood, couples experiencing infertility, or couples that have walked through miscarriage or loss of a child, you are uniquely positioned to help other childless women know that they aren't alone in this struggle.

Some of the sweetest conversations I've ever had are when I've been vulnerable and shared the difficulties I'm going through. Something happens when we are willing to expose the deepest parts of our souls with another . . . when we're willing to take off the mask and reveal that we don't have it all together, that we don't have all the answers, and that our lives are far from perfect. Perhaps the more precious interactions I've had are when I've been able to whisper into the lives of the hurting: "You're not alone." In those sacred moments, we get to remind fellow sufferers that we see them, we know them, and we love them.

I explained in earlier chapters that my mother was the first person I called in the midst of my loss. We both have experienced childlessness. Hers was infertility and a miscarriage, and mine was a missing uterus. Because our circumstances of childlessness were very different, I used to get upset when she told me she knew how I felt. Because I was much younger and saw myself as walking through this alone, I lashed out when my mom tried to comfort me. And because she had children, I felt her suffering had been redeemed while mine hadn't.

As time went on, we learned to better navigate our relationship. Communication became vital as we operated with different personalities and navigated different circumstances. I remember a conversation after she'd tried to comfort me, and I'd become upset. "Chelsea, I want so badly to be there for you! I can promise you that I'll never leave you, and that I'm committed to working through this with you." Does this not sound like the voice of our God? More important than anything my mom said or did, she was present. Don't ever underestimate the power of your presence.

My heart was also carrying more pain than I knew what to do with, and unfortunately, I chose to take it out on those closest to me. I wanted redemption on my time line, and when it didn't happen, I got angry. Don't be surprised if you encounter similar emotions in women you're ministering to, especially if the pain of their childlessness is new. Be careful when sharing your story that you don't overemphasize the similarity of your situations. The fact is you don't know exactly what someone else is going through. You don't know all the intimate details and emotional upheaval. Your role is to step up, and be present.

START A SUPPORT GROUP

Another way to harness the value of your story is by starting a support group for women walking through this journey. Perhaps you already know there are many women in your church or community who need such a resource. Consult your pastor, other key staff, or volunteers to find out the need and offer to facilitate a support gathering. It's important to make it broad enough that any woman struggling with childlessness can join. Discuss the different issues you're facing. Consider finding a Bible study or other biblical resource to work through together. Or simply provide a safe space where you can wrestle together with this hard story. Most important, pray together. There's nothing more powerful than a group of people gathered before the Lord, lifting their hurts and petitions up before a loving Father.

MAINTAIN A TENDER HEART

When you're no longer in the midst of a trial, it can be easy to forget the intensity of your feelings, especially if you're on the other side. Maybe your desire has been met, or maybe you've remained childless but have experienced healing. Time has a way of helping us begin to heal and readjust to life, regardless of our outcome. Sometimes the passing of time can cause us to forget the intensity of a trial. With this struggle in particular, it's critical to keep your heart tender, remembering people in your life who are still grieving. Our greatest goal and desire as Christians should be to help people know God or know Him better . . . to shepherd people toward a deeper and more intimate knowledge of Jesus.

Modeling for others the way our pain should propel us into His presence is a high calling. May we be a catalyst for men and women to learn to rest in God's love. Let this truth that C. S. Lewis so eloquently expresses in his book *The Problem of Pain* encourage you:

> For the far higher task of teaching fortitude and patience I was never fool enough to suppose myself qualified, nor have I anything to offer my readers except my conviction that when pain is to be borne, a little courage helps more than much knowledge, a little human sympathy more than much courage, and the least tincture of the love of God more than all.[6]

I continually find it helpful to remember that my childlessness doesn't define my entire life. Maybe the Lord will bless you with children one day, and maybe He won't. I implore you to keep your eyes fixed upon Him, love and serve others in your path, and don't waste your childlessness!

Before we proceed, join me in this prayer of submission:

Lord, I want to be used by You. I freely admit I don't always feel like choosing holiness instead of giving in to my desires. Sometimes I'd rather sit and wallow in my pain. While I know there is a time to grieve and to mourn, help me not to get stuck in my grief. I want to live a healthy and full life for You. I want my life to broadcast Your name for Your glory! Teach me how to do that in my moments and days. Show me how to obey You in the big and small things. Help me desire more of You. And Lord, I submit myself to Your will and ask You to please show me how to be a good steward of my story, even my childlessness.

REFLECTION & DISCUSSION

What are some practical ways you invite people into your life to see what God has done?

How can you begin sharing your stories and experiences with others?

Are you willing to start a support group for other childless women?

How do you see God's grace and love in this chapter?

EIGHT

HOW OUR COMMUNITIES CAN LOVE US WELL

Equipping the Church to Care for the Childless

*A*s I've walked through childlessness within the church community, I've been grateful for many Christian leaders, friends, and family who have supported me. But my experience hasn't been ideal, and I pray offering the following suggestions will help those in church— and other—leadership to better understand the trial of childlessness, to create an environment that encourages openness, and to more effectively reach out to the childless in their church family.

To my readers: This chapter will equip you by providing ideas and messages you can share with your pastor and other ministry leaders to equip them, in turn. (Sharing this book with them is another way!) I trust that you will add your own insights once you have reached a place of healing. From there, you can serve as a catalyst, or even a liaison, in your church community as it cultivates ways to minister to those suffering. Serving in such a role, however formally or informally, you can help your pastor, since most are faced with many needs from their congregations. If you are not yet in a place to aid or communicate more broadly with your church's leadership, I encourage you to meet with your pastor and let him know how the church community may be able to help care for you.

To our beloved church leaders: If you know someone walking the road of childlessness—perhaps this has been your own experience—you have an important opportunity to nurture and minister to women going through a tremendously difficult time. Though many Christians I've encountered obviously want to help, others shake their heads and say, "I'm so sorry." While I appreciate the sentiment, I desire to share some practical ways leaders and members of the church can help those wrestling with a deep longing for children. For those experiencing childlessness, it can be overwhelming to seek care. Conversely, those who would like to reach out may wonder: "What if I say or do the wrong thing? What if my words and actions are unintentionally hurtful?" Experiencing those feelings is completely normal but having the right tools to know how to properly care will help.

THE CHURCH'S ROLE

In my journey toward healing, the local church has been integral. When I moved to Washington, D.C., I immediately joined Capitol Hill Baptist Church where I began to learn firsthand how important the role of the church is in a Christian's life. I was raised attending church, but didn't personally grasp the importance of *planting* myself in a local church. The pastor at my church in D.C., Mark Dever, powerfully explains this in *What Is a Healthy Church?* "When a person becomes a Christian, he doesn't just join a local church because it's a good habit for growing in spiritual maturity. He joins a local church because it's the expression of what Christ has made him—a member of the body of Christ."[1]

Being part of a local church isn't simply about membership, it's about allowing yourself to be known and cared for. In Colossians, Paul gives a stunning snapshot of what we should be striving for as we care for one another:

> Put on then, as God's chosen ones, holy and beloved, compassionate hearts, kindness, humility, meekness, and patience, bearing with one another and, if one has a complaint against another, forgiving each other; as the Lord has forgiven you, so you also must forgive. And above all these put on love, which binds everything together in perfect harmony. And let the peace of Christ rule in your hearts, to which indeed you were called in one body. (Col. 3:12–15)

When Jesus walked the earth, He gave us the perfect example of what Paul was describing in those verses. We follow in His footsteps imperfectly, but we follow nevertheless. As important as it is for the church to step into the lives of the grieving, perfection isn't the goal. No one will ever perfectly love like Christ, but Christians have an opportunity to grow more like their Savior in how they respond to those suffering, including the childless.

Dear Pastor:
I have been part of a few churches that invite couples to the stage to announce that they are expecting. While we are called to rejoice with those who rejoice, the focus churches put on motherhood tends to alienate and hurt those unable to be mothers. I recognize that for pastors who are sensitive to this, even celebrating Mother's Day each year can feel like a balancing act. Year after year, I've sat in church with tears streaming down my cheeks as the entire service was focused on what I couldn't have. You want to honor mothers, but also be tender and sensitive to those longing for motherhood. Both can be achieved in such a service by recognizing mothers and cheering them on, but also providing other opportunities that give childless women in your congregation a voice.

In general, more often addressing topics such as infertility, miscarriage, and other forms of childlessness will both raise awareness of these issues and open doors for those suffering to share their trials. For instance, you might briefly mention these trials in a sermon about God's parental care or intentionally preach an entire sermon or sermon series dedicated to these topics.

These next sections offer additional suggestions for leaders and members of the church and beyond, so they may be better able to support those living with childlessness as well as the pastors who shepherd them.

PRAY FOR THE CHILDLESS

One of the most important things church communities can do for the childless is to regularly pray for them— *with* them and from the pulpit. What pastors choose to pray for on Sunday mornings teaches others *how* to pray and *what* to pray for. Here are some specific requests of those who need prayer:

> Pray that their hearts, souls, minds, and even bodies might be strengthened.

> Pray that they might know God's love through the compassion of fellow Christians.

> Pray that the Lord would answer their prayers for a child.

> Pray that they will use this trial to glorify the Lord.

> Pray that others might come to a saving knowledge of the Lord though this trial.

SUPPORT THEM AS THEY GRIEVE

Grief is a universal emotion, and every human has felt sorrow on some level. Yet it seems the prolonged grieving of others makes many people uncomfortable. Perhaps it's because we feel helpless when we can't quickly answer or solve a problem. If people can learn to lament, they must also learn how to comfort. Life is messy, so it's critical to learn how to sit in the discomfort with people.

My dear friend Karly, who has endured the trial of childlessness, offers this insightful guidance for those who wish to care for childless women:

> We are not looking for advice, but are just aching for prayers, companionship, compassion, and love. If at all possible, an effort should be made when you know that someone is facing such a terrible hardship. It is not your obligation to do anything, but I can tell you from firsthand experience that I will never forget those who reached out to us when we needed it the most, and I can also tell you that I completely regret not being that friend in the past. We tend to make things so hard—just simply go out and love someone. That's what they're looking for. It doesn't matter how. It just matters that you do.

As I finish this book, I'm preparing to walk down the aisle with Michael, the best man I've ever met. We met three years ago through a mutual friend and became fast friends ourselves. We spent time building that friendship, and Michael asked me out on a warm June evening after walking me home. I was elated. This handsome man I'd been crushing on asked me on a date! Fast forward a few months to early autumn, and as the weather cooled down, our relationship started to heat up.

Because we had a solid friendship, we began to have

some serious conversations early in our dating relationship. When I told Michael that I was barren, we were immediately thrown into a season of grief and struggle. I'd
had years to begin accepting my new reality, but Michael
was beginning the process of grieving for the first time.
A big struggle he encountered was that no one in his life
really knew what to do with his grief. My heart broke as
he was walked through a trying season, feeling like few
understood or knew what to say to properly comfort him.
Thankfully, as Michael began to share our struggle with
other men he trusted, he began to find comfort and solace.

If you walk away with just one thing from this final
chapter, it would be to offer to come alongside someone.
You don't have to have all the answers, and you don't need
formal training. Sometimes the most powerful thing you
can do is say, "I love you. I don't know all the 'right' things
to say, but I'm here for you. I want to learn how to care
well for your heart." It's an act of humility to confess this.

LEARN HOW TO ASK HELPFUL QUESTIONS

You give someone a great gift when you allow them to
grieve their loss. It takes humility not to force someone
to conform to your idea of what a grieving process should
look like. Everyone grieves differently and on a different
timetable, so women need to be given the freedom to take
the time they need to mourn the loss of their dream of
motherhood. We can't save someone out of their suffering; only the Lord can do that. A person's role in the life
of a sufferer is to show up and love with Christ's love.

Something that's been hugely beneficial for my heart
is when friends ask *how* I grieve. Since grief can take on

so many different forms, it's good to understand what's helpful and what's harmful for someone grieving. Below are a few questions to ask those who are suffering:

- Is it helpful for me to regularly ask how you're doing?
- Should I assume that you'll share your struggles when you're ready?
- How can I comfort you in your grief?
- What ways can I serve you?
- Are there particular things that trigger your grief?

For some people, asking them too often how they are doing can be hurtful, because it's a constant reminder of what they *don't* have and what they've lost. For others, if you avoid asking how they are (in an attempt not to hurt them), it can feel like you don't care enough to check in. Many hurt feelings can be avoided if open communication is practiced, even in the midst of the grieving. It might feel a bit awkward to ask for coaching on how to care for someone, but it's one of the most loving things you can do. Since humans are complex creatures, the way we feel comfort will vary widely.

AVOID USING BIBLE VERSES AS A QUICK FIX

God's Word is inerrant, full of power, wisdom, guidance, and comfort, but I've seen far too many people expect that a few moments of Bible reading will completely solve all of life's difficult circumstances. If we look through the pages of Scripture, we never see God tell us that His Word can instantly heal all our woes. Instead, we see again and again that He allows us to experience difficult seasons, often for longer than we'd like, because He knows that suffering shapes our character. One of the hurts I have experienced as I've walked through childlessness is when people, in an attempt to offer comfort, expected that by quoting a few Bible verses my heart would be instantly healed. Don't get me wrong, I adore the Word of God. Passages such as those in Psalm 119 have caused me to learn to love the Bible even more.

Yet, far too often, Christians attempt to provide comfort by offering a few verses, saying a quick prayer, and moving on. If Scripture doesn't offer a "quick fix" to grief or sorrow, why should we try to do so? Scripture should be used to shape every part of our lives and our hearts, but the actual work often takes more time than expected.

Many well-meaning friends have quoted verses such as Romans 8:28, which says that "we know that for those who love God all things work together for good, for those who are called according those his purpose." Those friends have expected me to instantly feel better and have been bewildered when that hasn't been the case. While verses like this hold truth, the truth can often take a long time to bear fruit.

Don't be so eager to help someone that you overlook what the Lord is already doing in their life. If they're still sorrowful after hearing a verse on God's goodness or sovereignty, don't criticize or doubt their faith. Mourning is a process. While you should definitely encourage the suffering with Scripture, allow them the time they need to process their pain.

DON'T ASSUME
THEY HAVE WEAK OR INSUFFICIENT FAITH

This was one of the most hurtful assumptions people made when they found out I couldn't have children. Many well-meaning friends tried to encourage me with the following admonishment: "Well, Chelsea, you never know what the Lord might do. Maybe you just need to trust Him more, pray more, have more faith." Everything in me wanted to scream, but most of the time I didn't feel like explaining the details of my childlessness. Instead, I'd smile and thank them for their thoughts. Having faith doesn't equal blessings from God. It's important to have good theology in this area.

Allow your beliefs about God's blessing and suffering to be challenged. Don't suggest that just because someone longs for children but doesn't have them, their relationship with God isn't right. God's ways are higher than ours, and sometimes He chooses the most faithful of His children to carry some of the heaviest burdens.

DON'T MINIMIZE
THE TRIAL OF CHILDLESSNESS

My heart broke as I listened to people share their bad experiences with friends and family who seemed to trivialize this struggle. Many may think they're being encouraging, but the advice or clichéd statements can come across as insensitive. Try not to assume that you have all the answers or that the woman you're attempting to comfort will be reassured by your own experience with suffering or childlessness. Rather than saying, "I know how you feel," it's more helpful to say, "I have been through a similar experience." Being willing to sit in the mystery of someone's suffering without offering an explanation is one of the greatest gifts you can give.

GET HER MIND OFF THE PROBLEM

Although I don't recommend practicing unhealthy escapism, it can be extremely helpful for those suffering to get their mind off their sorrows for a while. I suggest finding an occasional lighthearted conversation topic. Or suggest a new hobby, especially something creative. I'm not an artist, but I *adore* sitting down with a set of watercolors and can easily get lost in what I'm doing, temporarily escaping the pain.

TALK THROUGH THE PROBLEM

Sometimes it's therapeutic to talk out feelings and know you won't be judged for sharing how you actually feel. Talking doesn't erase the sorrow, but it helps release some built-up emotion. Don't hesitate to engage in conversation if a hurting woman wants to talk about her childlessness. Be willing to listen and ask constructive questions without offering answers or advice.

BE PRESENT

They are not expecting you to solve all their problems. A supportive way to care for people walking through childlessness is to simply be present and be available. Even if you haven't gone through a similar trial, be willing to listen and provide companionship.

Two of my closest friends, Rachel and Caroline, have modeled this so well for me. Hundreds of times, I've texted and called them as I continue to figure out what this childless journey looks like. Because grief is unpredictable, there were so many times when I'd just text them "Guys, I'm struggling," and immediately they'd respond with love, compassion, and encouragement. Never once did they make me feel like I'm too much trouble for them. I truly couldn't have written this book or continued to heal without their help!

There's a story in Exodus where we see Moses relying on Aaron and Hur to hold up his tired arms so the Israelites could prevail in battle (Ex. 17:8–13). Be the type of friend who will prop up someone when they get weak and tired. Sometimes, our souls are simply too exhausted, and we need people who help us when life gets to be too much to bear.

Be intentional in learning how your suffering friends best receive care. And don't be afraid to ask them outright, "What do you need in this moment? Would you like me to help get your mind off your struggle and think about something else? Would you like to talk through this some more?"

I highly recommend Dr. Gary Chapman's book *The 5 Love Languages* to help you determine the most effective way to give and receive love. When I'm going through something difficult, Michael always asks me, "Would it be more helpful if we talked this through right now or would you like to talk about something else?" It's such a helpful question because it prompts me to express what I need.

Michael isn't a mind reader and neither are you. No one is expecting you to respond perfectly every time or figure out exactly what they need in any given moment.

The weight of childlessness can be an overwhelming burden to bear, and it can also be a lot for others to help someone carry. While you have an important role to play in loving and supporting your struggling church member, friend, or family member, it's not your sole responsibility to always be there for them. The stronger their network of support, the less likely it is that individuals will burn out. Seek out elders, pastors, or other spiritual mentors to create a strong network and ensure that they'll be loved and cared for, even when you can't be there.

You can play such a powerful role in the lives of the childless. But remember, your responsibility is to point to God's fatherly care. Ultimately, it's His love, His hope, and His care for the childless that will heal their souls.

GOD IS REDEEMING A LEGACY OF LOSS AND LONGING

I've never met the woman who gave me life. However, Ana is often on my mind. I wonder about her. Has she married? Has she had more children? Is she happy? She's often the subject of my prayers, as I beg God to place people in her life who will tell her about His great love. I wonder if she thinks about me, her biological daughter, living on the other side of the ocean. We may never meet on earth, but she's played a large role in my life. Her selflessness as a teenager was beautiful, and I wouldn't be able to be sharing my story without her.

The irony of our stories isn't lost on me. She had a

child she couldn't keep; I long for a child I can't have. My adoptive mother couldn't birth children; yet, I grew up in a family full of children. All three of us women experienced childlessness; we all lost something.

But in and through the loss, the Lord has been redeeming all things to Himself. The greatest redemption has been getting to intimately know my Redeemer. Some people might view our three stories as tragic, since we've been denied motherhood for various reasons. I now see something different, something stunningly beautiful—the Lord's tender care of us.

What may look like a legacy of loss and longing pales in comparison to my adoption into the family of God. My physical adoption has taught me so much about my relationship with the Lord. From the beginning of my story—held by the woman who would unwittingly hand me over completely into God's care—until today, I can see the Lord's intentional love.

I never would have written my story this way; my struggle with childlessness is at times hard to bear. But in the struggles, the loneliness, and the longing, I've seen and experienced God's love in a way I don't think I would have if I hadn't gone through childlessness. I have learned how to say, "Not my will, but Yours be done" as I throw myself into the arms of a good and loving Father.

REFLECTION & DISCUSSION

What role can you play in equipping the church to care for the childless?

Have you shared your story with your pastor? If not, I encourage you to do so.

How can you put these suggestions into practice as you seek to care for other childless women?

How do you see God's grace and love in this chapter?

A FINAL NOTE
TO YOU, MY READER

When I look back over the past several years, I can see the Lord's hand guiding and working beyond my wildest imagination. Whether or not I felt it at the time, I am now aware of His care for me during every sleepless night, in the midst of every breakdown and every heartache, and even in the most unlikely places. My Father sees and knows me. And I've experienced healing as I've learned to see and know God.

Two weeks after completing the writing of this book, I celebrated my wedding day. Michael and I endured some hard seasons before realizing that joyous moment. Even though my childlessness has implications for how we one day start our family, Michael chose to unite his story with mine. I felt many fears over the years that I'd be rejected by a man because of my childlessness, but Michael put them all to rest. In his eyes, I'm not less of a woman— I'm *his* woman, the one he fell in love with, married, and started a new life with. My precious man is God's greatest gift to me on this side of heaven.

As I look back, I see redemption in my life. Sometimes, the Lord pulls back the curtain and shows us what redemption looks like. Yes, my childlessness will always be with me, but so will the hope I have in the Lord. Childlessness doesn't have to be the end of your story; God is at work, even in the most difficult circumstances. Instead, may you taste and see that the Lord is good, and even in the midst of your trial, may you experience the fullness of your Father's great love for you.

PRAYERS OF
LONGING AND HOPE

*W*hen we are grieving or angry or weary, we may find it difficult to put our emotions and requests into words. I know how that feels, and I know you do as well. In this book, I share the story of a small, picturesque chapel on the campus of my alma mater Liberty University. It was in that quiet chapel that I poured out prayers of lament and learned to persevere in hope. Below I offer several of those prayers, which are based on the book of Psalms. My prayer is that these words help you express your thoughts and emotions as you seek the hope that is found only in our all-knowing, all-powerful, and all-loving Father.

GRIEF

I am weary with my moaning; every night I flood my bed with tears; I drench my couch with my weeping. My eye wastes away because of grief (Ps. 6:6–7).

I will rejoice and be glad in your steadfast love,
because you have seen my affliction; you have
known the distress of my soul (Ps. 31:7).

Father, only You know the depth of my grief. I know because You wept at the tomb of Your friend Lazarus. Though I struggle to put my grief into words so that people understand, I'm thankful You have felt what I feel. I trust that You know the distress of my soul even when it seems grief and sorrow are my constant companions. And I know You are always with me. Thank You for walking this path with me and carrying me through it, as You "put my tears in your bottle" (Ps. 56:8).

ANGER

Refrain from anger, and forsake wrath! Fret not
yourself; it tends only to evil (Ps. 37:8).

Be angry and do not sin; do not let the sun go
down on your anger, and give no opportunity to
the devil (Eph. 4:26-27).

Jesus, today all of my pain is turning into anger . . . again. I confess that at times I have directed that anger toward my family, my friends, and even toward You. Forgive me. Help me to overcome this terrible emotion so that it will not turn to bitterness and cause me to sin. Please soften my heart and help me to trust in Your unfailing love.

COMFORT

*Even though I walk through the valley of the
shadow of death, I will fear no evil, for you are
with me; your rod and your staff, they comfort me*
(Ps. 23:4).

*Turn, O Lord, deliver my life; save me for the
sake of your steadfast love* (Ps. 6:4).

Jesus, my heart is heavy today and I need the sustaining
comfort only You can provide. Thank You for placing
loving people in my life who have tried to comfort me
in my grief. I do realize they care but sometimes they
inadvertently add to my sorrow and despair. Help me to
forgive them. And I ask you now in Your compassion to
provide me with comfort in my troubles. Help me to feel
encircled in Your eternal love, Father.

TRUST

*And those who know your name put their trust in
you, for you, O Lord, have not forsaken those
who seek you* (Ps. 9:10).

*But I have trusted in your steadfast love; my heart
shall rejoice in your salvation* (Ps. 13:5).

This journey is so hard, God. I often can't see purpose in
this trial . . . not clearly, anyway. I have questioned You a
lot and still do. I am learning, but please help me continue
to take my focus off of my pain, off of my circumstances,

and seek You instead. Give me eyes to see Your holiness, Your goodness, and Your faithfulness. Give me the strength and wisdom to trust You every moment.

(REDIRECTION OF) LONGING

"For your steadfast love is before my eyes, and I walk in your faithfulness" (Ps. 26:3).

"Rise up; come to our help! Redeem us for the sake of your steadfast love!" (Ps. 44:26).

Father, I believe I was "fearfully and wonderfully" (Ps. 139:14) made by You. Yet I long to be a mother. Redeem my unmet longing for a child, and make Your desires, my desires; make Your will, my will. Help me discern ways to redirect my love of children and my longing for motherhood toward other children and women who need to know they are loved and need to know Your love. I surrender to Your path and Your plan for my life.

PEACE

In peace I will both lie down and sleep; for you alone, O LORD, make me dwell in safety (Ps. 4:8).

O God, do not keep silence; do not hold your peace or be still, O God! (Ps. 83:1).

Lord, grant me Your peace. Although I often feel consumed by anxiety and inner turmoil, I know You have promised to give me peace. Please help me to cease my striving so I can experience peace as deep and constant as a river, peace that only comes from You. Help me to rest in the knowledge that You are my sovereign God and stead-fast Father.

HOPE

*Behold, the eye of the L*ORD *is on those who fear him, on those who hope in his steadfast love* (Ps. 33:18).

Let your steadfast love, O LORD, *be upon us, even as we hope in you* (Ps. 33:22).

Jesus, I feel overcome with hopelessness and it is becoming an impossible weight to carry. Yet I believe that through Your death and resurrection, You became my hope. Help me to remember Your great love for me and fill my heart with hope again. Because I know my hope is not found in the realization of my wants and dreams but in You alone.

FOR OTHERS

Father God, I know I am not the only person hurting because of my childlessness. It has affected my family and friends. And there are so many other women enduring the same trial. I ask you to comfort the women who aren't able to care for their children and must put them up for adoption. Sustain the single women who long to become mothers. Comfort the mothers who have lost a child to illness or accident or miscarriage. And be with women who are unable to conceive. You know our pain, and You know our hearts. Be with us, Lord. Bring us from a place of lament and longing to a place of everlasting hope in You. Amen.

30 SCRIPTURES TO SUSTAIN YOU IN THE MIDST OF CHILDLESSNESS

So she called the name of the Lord who spoke to her, "You are a God of seeing," for she said, "Truly here I have seen him who looks after me."
—Genesis 16:13

Know therefore that the Lord your God is God, the faithful God who keeps covenant and steadfast love *with those who love him and keep his commandments, to a thousand generations.*
—Deuteronomy 7:9 (niv)

It is the Lord who goes before you. He will be with you; he will not leave you or forsake you. Do not fear or be dismayed.
—Deuteronomy 31:8

No one will be able to stand against you all the days of your life. As I was with Moses, so I will be with you; I will never leave you nor forsake you.
—Joshua 1:5 (niv)

Then Job arose and tore his robe and shaved his head and fell on the ground and worshiped. And he said, "Naked I came from my mother's womb, and naked shall I return. The LORD gave, and the LORD has taken away; blessed be the name of the LORD."
—JOB 1:20

I lift up my eyes to the mountains—
where does my help come from?
My help comes from the LORD,
the Maker of heaven and earth.
—PSALM 121:1–2 (NIV)

Trust in the LORD with all your heart, and lean not on your own understanding; in all your ways acknowledge Him, and He will make straight your paths.
—PROVERBS 3:5–6

Surely he has borne our griefs and carried our sorrows.
—ISAIAH 53:4

I have loved you with an everlasting love;
therefore I have continued my faithfulness to you.
—JEREMIAH 31:3
Yet this I call to mind
and therefore I have hope:
Because of the LORD's great love we are not consumed,
for his compassions never fail.

They are new every morning;
great is your faithfulness.
I say to myself, "The LORD is my portion;
therefore I will wait for him."
The LORD is good to those whose hope is in him,
to the one who seeks him.
—LAMENTATIONS 3:21–25 (NIV)

The LORD your God is in your midst,
a mighty one who will save;
he will rejoice over you with gladness;
he will quiet you by his love;
he will exult over you with loud singing.
—ZEPHANIAH 3:17

Blessed are those who mourn, for they shall be
comforted.
—MATTHEW 5:4 (NIV)

And Jesus came and said to them, "All authority in
heaven and on earth has been given to me.... And behold,
I am with you always, to the end of the age."
—MATTHEW 28:18, 20
As the Father has loved me, so have I loved you. Abide in
my love. If you keep my commandments, you will abide
in my love, just as I have kept my Father's commandments
and abide in his love. These things I have spoken to you,

that my joy may be in you, and that your joy may be full.
—JOHN 15:9–11

Therefore, since we have been justified by faith, we have
peace with God through our Lord Jesus Christ. Through
him we have also obtained access by faith into this
grace in which we stand, and we rejoice in hope of
the glory of God. Not only that, but we rejoice in our
sufferings, knowing that suffering produces endurance,
and endurance produces character, and character produces hope, and hope does not put us to shame, because
God's love has been poured into our hearts through the
Holy Spirit who has been given to us.
—ROMANS 5:1–5

In all these things we are more than conquerors through
him who loved us. For I am convinced that neither death
nor life, neither angels nor demons, neither the present
nor the future, nor any powers, neither height nor depth,
nor anything else in all creation, will be able to separate us
from the love of God that is in Christ Jesus our Lord.
—ROMANS 8:37–39 (NIV)

May the God of hope fill you with all joy and peace as
you trust in him, so that you may overflow with hope by
the power of the Holy Spirit.
—ROMANS 15:13 (NIV)
Praise be to the God and Father of our Lord Jesus
Christ, the Father of compassion and the God of all
comfort, who comforts us in all our troubles, so that we
can comfort those in any trouble with the comfort we

ourselves receive from God.
—2 CORINTHIANS 1:3-4 (NIV)

Therefore we do not lose heart. Though outwardly we
are wasting away, yet inwardly we are being renewed
day by day. For our light and momentary troubles are
achieving for us an eternal glory that far outweighs them
all. So we fix our eyes not on what is seen, but on what
is unseen, since what is seen is temporary, but what is
unseen is eternal.
—2 CORINTHIANS 4:16–18 (NIV)

But he said to me, "My grace is sufficient for you, for
my power is made perfect in weakness." Therefore I will
boast all the more gladly about my weaknesses, so that
Christ's power may rest on me. That is why, for Christ's
sake, I delight in weaknesses, in insults, in hardships, in
persecutions, in difficulties. For when I am weak, then I
am strong.
—2 CORINTHIANS 12:9–10 (NIV)

Bear one another's burdens, and so fulfill the law of Christ.
—GALATIANS 6:2

But because of his great love for us, God, who is rich in
mercy, made us alive with Christ even when we were dead
in transgressions—it is by grace you have been saved.
—EPHESIANS 2:4–5 (NIV)
I have learned in whatever situation I am to be content. I
know how to be brought low, and I know how to abound.
In any and every circumstance, I have learned the secret of
facing plenty and hunger, abundance and need. I can do all

things through him who strengthens me.
—PHILIPPIANS 4:11–13

And my God will meet all your needs according to the
riches of his glory in Christ Jesus.
—PHILIPPIANS 4:19 (NIV)

Put on then, as God's chosen ones, holy and beloved,
compassionate hearts, kindness, humility, meekness, and
patience, bearing with one another and, if one has a com-
plaint against another, forgiving each other; as the Lord
has forgiven you, so you also must forgive. And above
all these put on love, which binds everything together
in perfect harmony. And let the peace of Christ rule in
your hearts, to which indeed you were called in one body.
And be thankful.
—COLOSSIANS 3:12–15

Rejoice always, pray continually, give thanks in
all circumstances; for this is God's will for you in
Christ Jesus.
—1 THESSALONIANS 5:16-18 (NIV)

For we do not have a high priest who is unable to sympa-
thize with our weaknesses, but one who in every respect
has been tempted as we are, yet without sin. Let us then
with confidence draw near to the throne of grace, that we

may receive mercy and find grace to help in time of need.
—HEBREWS 4:15–16

Let us run with perseverance the race marked out for us, fixing our eyes on Jesus, the pioneer and perfecter of faith.
—HEBREWS 12:1–2 (NIV)

Beloved, do not be surprised at the fiery trial when it comes upon you to test you, as though something strange were happening to you. But rejoice insofar as you share Christ's sufferings, that you may also rejoice and be glad when his glory is revealed.
—1 PETER 4:12–13

Behold, the dwelling place of God is with man. He will dwell with them, and they will be his people, and God himself will be with them as their God. He will wipe away every tear from their eyes, and death shall be no more, neither shall there be mourning, nor crying, nor pain anymore, for the former things have passed away.
—REVELATION 21:2–4

NOTES

Introduction

1. Karen Breslau, "Overplanned Parenthood: Ceaușescus cruel law," *Newsweek*, January 22, 1990, 35.
2. Vlad Odobescu, "Half a million kids survived Romania's 'slaughterhouses of souls.' Will they ever heal?" *The Week*, January 17, 2016, http://theweek.com/articles/597406/half-million-kids-survived-romanias-slaughterhouses-souls-ever-heal.

Chapter 1: The Silent Struggle

1. Mayo Clinic Staff, "Panic attacks and panic disorders," Mayo Clinic, http://www.mayoclinic.org/diseases-conditions/panic-attacks/basics/definition/con-20020825.
2. "Key Statistics from the National Survey of Family Growth," Centers for Disease Control and Prevention, August 14, 2017, https://www.cdc.gov/nchs/nsfg/key_statistics.htm.
3. Catherine Pearson, "Miscarriage Causes, Rates Widely Misunderstood, Study Shows," *Huffington Post*, October 17, 2013, http://www.huffingtonpost.com/2013/10/17/miscarriage-cause_n_4116712.html.
4. "Miscarriage Statistics Week-By-Week: Risks & Signs," *Check Pregnancy*, August 23, 2015, https://www.checkpregnancy.com/miscarriage-statistics/.
5. Catherine Pearson, "Miscarriage Causes, Rates Widely Misunderstood, Study Shows," *Huffington Post*, October 17, 2013, http://www.huffingtonpost.com/2013/10/17/miscarriage-cause_n_4116712.html.
6. Harvard Medical School, "The psychological impact of infertility and its treatment," *Harvard Health Publishing*, May 2009, https://www.health.harvard.edu/newsletter_article/The-psychological-impact-of-infertility-and-its-treatment.
7. Harvard Medical School, "Takotusbo cardiomyopathy (broken-heart syndrome), *Harvard Health Publishing*, November 2010, Updated April 6, 2016, https://www.health.harvard.edu/heart-health/takotsubo-cardiomyopathy-broken-heart-syndrome.
8. Elisabeth Elliot, *Let Me Be a Woman* (Carol Stream, IL: Tyndale House, 1976), 8.
9. Carolyn Mahaney, Nicole Whitacre, *True Beauty* (Wheaton, IL: Crossway, 2014), 81.
10. Michael Card, *A Sacred Sorrow: Reaching Out to God in the Lost Language of Lament* (Colorado Springs: NavPress, 1994), 32.

Chapter 2: Seasons of Sorrow

1. Carol Kent, *He Holds My Hand: Experiencing God's Presence and Protection* (Carol Stream, IL: Tyndale House, 2017), June 11 entry.

2. Dr. John Rippon, "How Firm a Foundation," 1787, https://www.hymnal.net/en/hymn/h/339.

3. John Piper, "Insanity and Spiritual Songs in the Soul of a Saint, Reflections on the Life of William Cowper," *Desiring God*, January 29, 1992, http://www.desiringgod.org/messages/insanity-and-spiritual-songs-in-the-soul-of-a-saint.

4. Michael Card, *A Sacred Sorrow: Reaching Out to God in the Lost Language of Lament* (Colorado Springs: NavPress, 2005), 29.

5. David Qaoud, "Charles Spurgeon on the Sweet Sovereignty of God," *Gospel Relevance*, June 22, 2015, http://gospelrelevance.com/2015/06/22/charles-spurgeon-on-the-sovereignty-of-god/.

6. Jerry Bridges, *Trusting God* (Colorado Springs: NavPress, 2008), 16.

7. Will Kynes, "God's Grace in the Old Testament: Considering the *Hesed* of the Lord," Knowing and Doing, a newsletter from C. S. Lewis Institute, Summer 2010, http://www.cslewisinstitute.org/webfm_send/430.

8. Charles Spurgeon, *Morning and Evening* (Wheaton, IL: Crossway 2003), March 18, evening.

Chapter 3: Trusting God's No

1. D. A. Carson, *How Long, O Lord?: Reflections on Suffering and Evil* (Grand Rapids, MI: Baker Academic, 2006), 66.

2. Stephen J. Nichols, *Bonhoeffer on the Christian Life: From the Cross, for the World* (Wheaton, IL: Crossway, 2013), 160.

3. Albert Y. Hsu, *Grieving a Suicide: A Loved One's Search for Comfort, Answers, and Hope* (Westmont, IL: InterVarsity, 2002), 41.

4. Nancy Guthrie, "What Grieving People Wish You Knew at Christmas," *Desiring God*, December 21, 2016, http://www.desiringgod.org/articles/what-grieving-people-wish-you-knew-at-christmas.

5. Jean E. Jones, "The Journey of Childlessness," *Today's Christian Woman*, April 2010, http://www.todayschristianwoman.com/articles/2010/april/journeychildlessness.html.

6. Vaneetha Rendall Risner, "Job and the Prosperity Gospel," May 28, 2015, http://danceintherain.com/2015/05/28/job-and-the-prosperity-gospel/.

7. Timothy Keller, *Jesus the King: Understanding the Life and Death of the Son of God* (New York: Penguin Books, 2013), 58.

8. Charles H. Spurgeon, "A Wonderful Transformation," No. 2983, A Sermon Published on Thursday, April 12, 1906. Delivered

by C. H. Spurgeon at the Metropolitan Tabernacle, Newington, October 3, 1875, http://www.spurgeongems.org/vols52-54 /chs2983.pdf.

Chapter 4: Grieving Your Unfulfilled Desire

1. John MacArthur and ESV Bibles by Crossway, *The MacArthur Study Bible* (Wheaton, IL: Crossway, 2013), 377.
2. Winfred O. Neely, "1 Samuel," in *The Moody Bible Commentary*, Michael Rydelnik and Michael Vanlaningham, eds. (Chicago: Moody, 2014), 404.
3. Linda Lawrence Hunt, "3 Myths about Grief," The Christian Century, August 17, 2015, https://www.christiancentury.org /blogs/archive/2015-07/3-myths-about-grief.
4. Lisa Podgurski, M.D., "How Long Is Too Long? Complicated Grief," Palliative Care Case of the Month, Vol. 14, No. 42, December 2014.
5. Doris Dahdouh, "This Is What Happens to Your Body When You Suppress Your Emotions," FitLife.tv, http://fitlife.tv/ this-is-what-happens-to-your-body-when-you-suppress-your-emotions-original/.
6. Daniel Goleman, "Study of Normal Mourning Process Illuminates Grief Gone Awry," *The New York Times,* March 29, 1988, http://www.nytimes.com/1988/03/29/science/study-of-normal-mourning-process-illuminates-grief-gone-awry. html?pagewanted=all&mcubz=1.
7. Christina Fox, "Helping the Hurting," November 5, 2014, The Gospel Coalition, https://www.thegospelcoalition.org/article /helping-hurting.
8. Donald S. Whitney, *Spiritual Disciplines for the Christian Life* (Colorado Springs: NavPress, 2014), 6.
9. Timothy Keller, *Prayer: Experiencing Awe and Intimacy with God* (New York: Penguin Books, 2016), 55–56.
10. Corrie ten Boom with Elizabeth and John Sherrill, *The Hiding Place* (Grand Rapids, MI: Chosen Books, 2006), 209–10.

Chapter 5: We Have This Hope!

1. Merriam-Webster Dictionary online, https://www.merriam-webster.com/dictionary/hope.
2. Julie Clinton, *Becoming a Woman of Extraordinary Faith: What If You Gave It All to God?* (Eugene, OR: Harvest House, 2011) 26.
3. D. Martyn Lloyd-Jones, *Spiritual Depression: Its Causes and Cures* (Grand Rapids: Eerdmans, 1965), 21.
4. Rachel Pate, "Why Does God Call Us Sheep," *In Honor of the King*, April 16, 2011, http://inhonoroftheking.blogspot. com/2011/04/why-does-god-call-us-sheep.html.

5. Charles Dyer with Eva Rydelnik, "1 Samuel," in *The Moody Bible Commentary*, Michael Rydelnik and Michael Vanlaningham, eds. (Chicago: Moody, 2014), 1189.
6. Lindsay Terry, "The Story Behind the Song: It Is Well," *The St. Augustine Record*, January 27, 2017, http://staugustine.com /living/religion/2014-10-16/story-behind-song-it-well-my-soul.
7. John Piper, *Desiring God*, April 19, 2014, https://www.youtube .com/watch?v=r5kUSkm0wis.
8. C. S. Lewis, *The Four Loves* (New York: HarperOne, 2017), 121.

Chapter 6: Ways to Live Out the Longing

1. Kelly Minter, "A Disney Trip and 3 Reasons I'm Choosing Aunthood," November 21, 2016, http://kellyminter.com/disney-trip-3-reasons-im-choosing-aunthood/.
2. "Orphans," UNICEF, June 16, 2017, https://www.unicef.org /media/media_45279.html.
3. "Where Do Orphans Come From?" World Orphans, November 17, 2016, https://www.worldorphans.org/featured-articles/2016/11/17/where-do-orphans-come-from.
4. Louis Gilman and Susan Freivalds, "Choosing adoption: Cost, benefits, and the risk of the main options," Babycenter, March 2017, https://www.babycenter.com/0_choosing-adoption-cost-benefits-and-risk-of-the-main-options_1373536.b.
5. Emma Davis, "Curious about adopting from foster care? Here's what it's really like," *Today*, December 2, 2015, https://www.today.com/parents/family-all-my-own-why-adopting-foster-care-easier-it-t34871
6. John Piper, "Adoption: The Heart of the Gospel," *Desiring God*, February 10, 2007, http://www.desiringgod.org/messages/adoption-the-heart-of-the-gospel.
7. Jen Christensen, "Record Number of Women Using IVF to Get Pregnant," CNN, February 18, 2014, http://www.cnn.com/2014/02/17/health/record-ivf-use/index.html.
8. Michaeleen Doucleff, "IVF Baby Boom: Births from Fertility Procedures Hit New High," NPR, February 18, 2014, http://www.npr.org/sections/health-shots/2014/02/18/279035110/ivf-baby-boom-births-from-fertility-procedure-hit-new-high.
9. "In Vitro Fertilization (IVF)," AmericanPregnancy.org, http://americanpregnancy.org/infertility/in-vitro-fertilization/.
10. Beth A. Malizia and Michele R. Hacker, "Cumulative Live-Birth Rates after In Vitro Fertilization," Boston IVF, January 15, https://www.bostonivf.com/content/editor/MDPublications/Penzias-Cumulative-live-birth-rates-after-in-vitro-fertilization-2009.pdf.
11. "The Cost of Infertility Treatment," Resolve, The National Infertility Association, Summer 2006, http://www.resolve.org

/family-building-options/making-treatment-affordable/the-costs-of-infertility-treatment.html?referrer=https://www.google.com/.

12. "Abortion Viewed in Moral Terms: Fewer See Stem Cell Research and IVF as Moral Issues," Pew Research Center, August 15, 2013, http://www.pewforum.org/2013/08/15/abortion-viewed-in-moral-terms/.

13. Bernice Yeung and Jonathan Jones, "When pregnancy dreams become IVF nightmares," Reveal News, June 1, 2017, https://www.revealnews.org/article/when-pregnancy-dreams-become-ivf-nightmares/.

14. "Embryo Adoption," Health and Human Services," August 3, 2017, https://www.hhs.gov/opa/about-opa/embryo-adoption/index.html.

15. Shane Pruitt, "Does In Vitro Fertilization Undermine Sanctity of Life?" *Christian Post*, March 15, 2016, http://www.christianpost.com/news/in-vitro-fertilization-undermine-sanctity-of-life-pregnancy-babies-abortion-158569/.

16. "Anticipated Costs (Of Surrogacy)," Agency for Surrogacy Solutions, Inc., https://www.surrogacysolutionsinc.com/intended-parents/anticipated-costs/.

Chapter 7: Don't Waste Your Childlessness

1. John Piper, *Don't Waste Your Life* (Wheaton, IL: Crossway, 2003), 12–13.

2. Matthew Henry, *An Exposition of the Old and New Testament* (Philadelphia: Haswell, Barrington & Haswell Publisher, 1706), 485.

3. Timothy Keller, *Walking with God through Pain and Suffering* (New York: Penguin Group, 2013), 9.

4. A. W. Tozer, *The Best of A. W. Tozer, Book One* (Chicago: Moody, 2000), 179.

5. Ann Voskamp, *The Broken Way—A Daring Path into the Abundant Life* (Grand Rapids: Zondervan, 2016), 41.

6. C. S. Lewis, *The Problem of Pain* (New York: Harper Collins, 1940), xii.

Chapter 8: How Our Communities Can Love Us Well

1. Mark Dever, *What Is a Healthy Church?* (Wheaton, IL: Crossway, 2007), 26.

RECOMMENDED RESOURCES

BOOKS

Adopted for Life by Russell Moore

Don't Waste Your Life by John Piper

Just Show Up by Kara Tippetts and Jill Buteyn

Outside the Womb: Moral Guidance for Assisted Reproduction by Scott Rae and Joy Riley

A Sacred Sorrow by Michael Card

Suffering and the Sovereignty of God by John Piper

Walking with God through Pain and Suffering by Timothy Keller

ADOPTION ASSISTANCE INFORMATION

www.adoptionassistance.com

www.bethany.org

www.davethomasfoundation.com

www.fundyouradoption.org

www.giftofadoption.com

Note: Some employers provide forms of adoption assistance. Be sure to talk with them and see what kind of help they can offer.

ACKNOWLEDGMENTS

I was terrified to write this book. Baring my soul to the world felt scary, and I considered backing out multiple times. When I first started writing, I felt as if I was standing at the base of a mountain, not sure if I'd ever make it to the top. The journey has been difficult and exhausting, but it has been deeply worth it. I've been compelled to keep going, because I desperately desire other childless women to know they have comfort in the midst of the sorrow. My prayer is that this book will serve the souls of many. The words "thank you" seem to fall short of expressing my gratitude, but I will use them nevertheless.

To the childless women. This book is my love letter to you. How I wish I could come and spend time with each one of you, hug you, cry, and pray with you. I've had the honor of getting to know many of you, with different experiences of childlessness. Each story is so precious to me. More importantly, it's precious to our Father. Thank you for teaching me. May we unite together in a beautiful sisterhood that supports one another in our dark seasons.

To the love of my life, Michael. Thank you for being willing to join your story with mine. Thank you for self-lessly loving me as I've written this book. You are my joy and my treasure.

To my family. You are the people who know me the best and have loved me the longest. I can never thank you enough for all you've done for me. The most important thing you've ever done is introducing me to Christ and teaching me how to be His child.

To Rachel Wear, Caroline Biggs, Amanda Sanders. Words cannot begin to tell you how grateful I am for your friendship. Thank you for being "my people," my first call, for loving me with the purest love, and for always pointing me to Christ. I'm forever changed because of your friendship. You've helped shape me into the woman I am today.

To all the people who entered into my suffering with me. Arielle Able, Melanie Andruzzi, Joylane Barton, Sarah Bradshaw, Anna Cribb, Bethany Cummings, Angela Edge, Ken Farnaso, Lauren Moore, Ericka Morris, Danielle Napieralski, Alexandria Paolozzi, Kristi Peterson, Lindsey Sobolik, Liz Sobolik, Mike Sobolik, and Morgan Stone. Your love and support mean more to me than you'll ever know. Words cannot begin to tell you how grateful I am for your friendship. Thank you for walking this journey with me. Thank you for listening to me. Thank you for loving me.

To Adam Dalton. I'm so glad I "happened" to meet you on that hot August day at a conference. Thank you for listening to my idea, believing in my message, and providing encouragement along the way.

To Ingrid Beck and Amanda Cleary Eastep. Thank you for shaping this book into what it is today. You both walked through long weeks of editing and were incredibly kind and patient to me. The book was in the most capable hands, and I am forever grateful.

CAN GOD'S LOVE HURT?

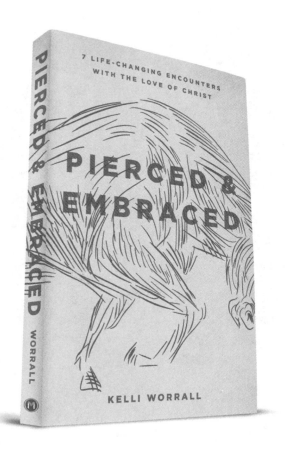

Pierced & Embraced digs deeply into seven encounters that Jesus had with a wide variety of women in the Gospels to show how His love can be just as powerful in our lives today. It mixes attentive scriptural engagement with contemporary research and personal narrative, making the content accessible, engaging, and practical.

978-0-8024-1631-5 | also available as an eBook

SUFFERING IS A SEASON.
HOPE IS ETERNAL.

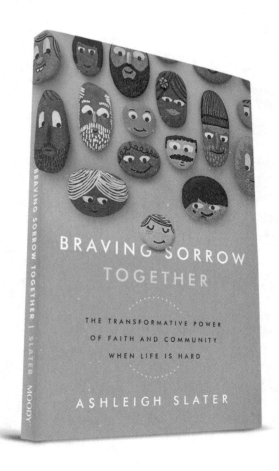

Braving Sorrow Together examines the nature of grief and loss in several universal arenas, such as relationships, health, career, and the home. For anyone who ever struggles—and that's all of us—*Braving Sorrow Together* will teach us to move through trials with wisdom, releasing anxiety and receiving the help and comfort God so bountifully provides.

978-0-8024-1659-9 | also available as an eBook

LIVING FREELY IN A CULTURE OF COMPARISON

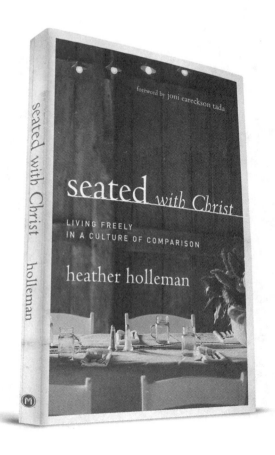

Seated with Christ is for anyone tired of comparing, competing, and clamoring for acceptance. In elegant, vulnerable prose, English lecturer Heather Holleman unveils the wonder of our being seated with Christ in the heavens (Eph. 2:6). This reflective journey into Scripture inspires us to live as we were meant to: freely and securely.

978-0-8024-1343-7 | also available as an eBook

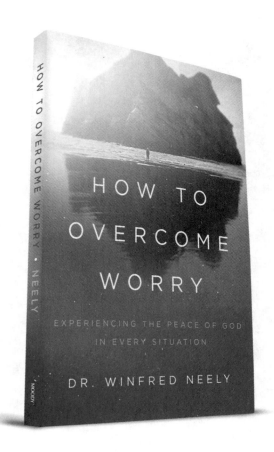